Living a Fulfilling Life with Scleroderma

A Healthy Eating Plan to Reduce Inflammation, Alleviate Symptoms of Systemic Sclerosis, Support Skin and Tissue Health

DR LANA BROWN, RN

Copyright Page

Table of Contents

CHAPTER I

SCLERODERMA AND ITS IMPACT ON NUTRITION

What is Scleroderma?

Scleroderma (sklair-oh-DUR-muh), also known as systemic sclerosis, is a group of rare diseases that involve the hardening and tightening of the skin i.e. your body produce tissue that's thicker than it should be. As a result, your skin gets thick and tight, and scars can form on your lungs and kidneys. Your blood vessels may thicken and stop working the way they should. This leads to tissue damage and high blood pressure.

Scleroderma usually affects your skin, but can cause symptoms in any tissue throughout your body.

Scleroderma also may cause problems in the blood vessels, internal organs and digestive tract.

Scleroderma is an autoimmune disorder. Autoimmune disorders happen when your immune system accidentally attacks your body instead of protecting it. Experts don't know why your immune system turns on you. It's like it can no longer tell the difference between what's healthy and what's not — between what's you and what's an invader like bacteria or a virus.

If you have scleroderma, your immune system triggers your body's cells to produce too much collagen (a protein). Your body needs collagen to have strong, healthy connective tissue to support your organs and hold parts of your body in place. But when you produce too much of it, your skin and other tissue can be thicker and more fibrous than they should be.

Scleroderma is a chronic condition, which means you'll need to manage your symptoms for a long time (maybe the rest of your life). It can also cause life-threatening complications if it affects tissue in your organs.

Scleroderma is often categorized as limited or diffuse, which refers only to the degree of skin involvement. Both types can involve any of the other vascular or organ symptoms that are part of the disease. Localized scleroderma, also known as morphea, affects only the skin.

While there is no cure for scleroderma, treatments can ease symptoms, slow progression and improve quality of life.

Scleroderma commonly affects people 30 to 50 years of age but is found in all ages. Also, women are typically more likely than men to receive a diagnosis of this condition.

Systemic sclerosis vs. scleroderma

Systemic sclerosis is also called systemic scleroderma. It's another form of scleroderma that can affect many organ systems in your body. It's more serious than localized scleroderma, which tends to only affect your skin and the structures that underlie your skin, such as fat, ligaments, and tendons.

In addition to affecting your skin, systemic sclerosis may also affect your blood vessels and other internal organs, such as your heart, lungs, and kidneys.

How common is scleroderma?

Scleroderma is rare. Experts estimate that all types of scleroderma affect around 250 out of every 1 million people in the U.S. Around 100,000 people in the U.S. have systemic scleroderma.

Causes

Scleroderma happens when the body produces too much collagen and it builds up in body tissues. Collagen is a fibrous type of protein that makes up the body's connective tissues, including the skin.

Experts don't know exactly what causes this process to begin, but the body's immune system appears to play a role. Most likely, scleroderma is caused by a combination of factors, including immune system problems, genetics and environmental triggers.

Risk factors

Anyone can get scleroderma, but it is more common in people assigned female at birth. People typically get scleroderma between ages 30 and 50. Black people often have earlier onset and are more likely to have more skin involvement and lung disease.

Several other combined factors appear to influence the risk of having scleroderma:

• **Genetics**. People who have certain gene changes appear to be more likely to develop scleroderma. This may explain why scleroderma appears to run in families in a small number of people and why some types of scleroderma are more common for people in certain racial and ethnic groups.

• **Environmental triggers**. Research suggests that in some people, scleroderma symptoms may be triggered by exposure to certain viruses, medicines or drugs. Repeated exposure, such as at work, to certain harmful substances or chemicals also may increase the risk of scleroderma. An environmental trigger is not identified for most people.

• **Immune system conditions**. Scleroderma is believed to be an autoimmune disease. This means that it occurs in part because the body's immune system begins to attack the connective tissues. People who have scleroderma also may have symptoms of another autoimmune disease such as rheumatoid arthritis, lupus or Sjogren syndrome.

Complications

Scleroderma complications range from mild to serious and can affect the:

Fingertips. In systemic sclerosis, Raynaud's phenomenon can become so severe that the restricted blood flow permanently damages the tissue at the fingertips, causing pits or skin sores. In some people, the tissue on the fingertips may die.

Lungs. Scarring of lung tissue can impact the ability to breathe and tolerance for exercise. High blood pressure in the arteries to the lungs also may happen.

Kidneys. A serious kidney complication, called scleroderma renal crisis, involves a sudden increase in blood pressure and rapid kidney failure. Prompt treatment of this condition is important to preserve kidney function.

Heart. Scarring of heart tissue increases the risk of irregular heartbeats and heart failure. Scleroderma also can cause inflammation of the sac surrounding the heart.

Teeth. Serious tightening of facial skin can cause the mouth to become smaller and narrower. This may make it hard to brush the teeth or to have them professionally cleaned or restored. People who have scleroderma often don't make typical amounts of saliva, so the risk of dental decay increases even more.

Digestive system. Digestive complications of scleroderma can include heartburn and difficulty swallowing. Scleroderma also can cause bouts of cramps, bloating, constipation or diarrhea. Some people who have scleroderma also may have problems absorbing nutrients due to overgrowth of bacteria in the intestine.

Joints. The skin over joints can become so tight that it restricts flexibility and movement, particularly in the hands.

Gangrene. In extreme cases, abnormal or narrowed blood vessels combined with severe Raynaud's can lead to gangrene and may necessitate amputation.

Incontinence. Weakening of the sphincter muscles and/or abnormal gastrointestinal motility can lead to stool incontinence.

Types of Scleroderma and Their Symptoms

Types of Scleroderma

The two main categories of scleroderma include:

• **Localized scleroderma**, which affects the skin and occasionally the underlying muscles or joints

• **Systemic sclerosis,** which involves blood vessels and internal organs throughout the body

Localized scleroderma affects mostly children and is less severe than systemic sclerosis, which is more common in adults. The causes of scleroderma are still unknown, but it is believed to be related to a buildup of collagen (a protein in connective tissue) in the skin and an abnormal immune system response.

Localized scleroderma may appear in one spot or in several patches or regions of the skin. It has the following two main subtypes.

• **Linear scleroderma:** Lesions look like straight lines or streaks.

• **Morphea scleroderma**: Reddish oval patches form.

Common Symptoms of Localized Scleroderma

Localized scleroderma is a rare condition. Linear scleroderma typically involves both the surface and deeper layers of the skin, but morphea scleroderma doesn't tend to go beyond the surface layers of the epidermis and dermis.

Linear Scleroderma

Linear scleroderma forms into lines as it hardens. It often occurs on one side of the body and can appear as a line down an arm or leg, or sometimes the head. As it spreads to deeper skin layers, it may also involve muscle and bone. Linear scleroderma typically occurs in children.

Common symptoms of linear scleroderma include:

• Lines or streaks of hardened, waxy skin on the trunk and limbs or face and scalp

• Skin discoloration that may appear lighter or darker

• Joint tightness

Morphea Scleroderma

Morphea scleroderma, the more common form of localized scleroderma, most often forms on the abdomen and back. It can also sometimes develop on the face, arms, and legs.

Morphea scleroderma can be limited to one to four small patches (plaque morphea) or in some cases it can spread over large areas of the body (generalized morphea). It most commonly occurs in adults between the ages of o and o, but can also occur in children.

Common symptoms include:

• Patches of reddish skin that thicken into firm, oval-shaped areas on the abdomen, chest, or back

• Skin becomes waxy and shiny as it tightens

• Center of the patches can be ivory or yellow with violet borders

• Pruritis (itchy skin)

Morphea scleroderma tends to be oval and reddish, but the waxy patches may vary in color, shade (light or dark), size, and shape. The patches may get larger or shrink, and they may disappear spontaneously.

Localized scleroderma typically goes away over time, but it may leave skin discoloration even after it resolves. Linear scleroderma typically lasts two to five years, and morphea lesions last an average of three to five years.

Common Symptoms of Systemic Sclerosis

Systemic sclerosis (SSc) can affect connective tissues in many parts of the body. The two main subtypes are limited cutaneous SSc, which progresses slowly over a period of years, and diffuse cutaneous SSc, which covers more skin area and progresses more quickly to multiple organs and systems.

Limited Cutaneous Systemic Sclerosis

Limited cutaneous SSc is also called CREST syndrome, an acronym for its common conditions and symptoms.

CREST syndrome

People with limited cutaneous SSc may have two or more common features of CREST syndrome:

• **Calcinosis**, which are calcium deposits in the skin

• **Raynaud's phenomenon**, a spasm of blood vessels in response to cold, stress, or emotional upset that can decrease blood flow in fingers or toes

• **Esophageal dysfunction**, which is when smooth muscles that line the esophagus lose normal movement and function

• **Sclerodactyly**, a thickening and tightening of the skin of the fingers and hands

• **Telangiectasia,** a swelling of capillaries (small blood vessels) near the surface of the skin on the face and hands that causes red spots

Common skin-related symptoms of limited cutaneous SSc include:

• Fingers or toes that turn blue and/or white when cold and then become bright red when warmed back up

• Swelling and sausage-like appearance of fingers

• Skin thickening on the face, arms, and legs

• Small, hard lumps in or under the skin (calcinosis)

• Fingers curl due to skin tightening

• Reduced range of finger motion

• Waxy, mask-like appearance of the face

• Tiny red spots on hands and face

• Abnormal skin dryness

An estimated 95% of SSc cases begin with Raynaud's phenomenon. In limited cutaneous SSc, Raynaud's phenomenon often occurs for several years prior to skin thickening.

Early symptoms of limited cutaneous SSc involve sensitivity and/or swelling of fingers or toes. The swelling of the hands may be especially pronounced in the morning due to muscle inactivity during sleeping hours. Fingers may look sausage-like, making it difficult to close the hand into a fist. Symptoms may subside as the day goes on.

Gastrointestinal issues affect up to 0% of people who have SSc. The esophagus is the most commonly involved organ, affecting % of people with SSc. The symptoms are due to structural and functional changes of the esophagus that can occur in limited or diffuse cutaneous SSc.

Common esophageal symptoms include:

• Heartburn (the sensation of burning behind the breast bone)

• Difficulty or pain while swallowing

• Regurgitation

• Hoarseness

• Mouth ulcers

• Acid taste in the mouth

The most common symptom is heartburn. This is due to irritation of the esophagus by acid reflux (stomach acid backing up or refluxing up the esophagus).

Sometimes excess collagen collects in the tissue between the lungs' air sacs in people with limited cutaneous SSc, making the lung tissue stiffer and less able to work properly. If the lungs become affected, common additional symptoms include:

• Persistent cough

• Shortness of breath

Diffuse Cutaneous Systemic Sclerosis

Raynaud's phenomenon often occurs simultaneously or just prior to skin thickening in those with diffuse cutaneous SSc. Diffuse cutaneous SSc can involve the heart, lungs, kidneys, gastrointestinal tract, and central and peripheral nervous systems.

Common symptoms of diffuse cutaneous SSc include:

• Swelling and sausage-like appearance of fingers

• Skin thickening over large areas of the torso, hands, arms, and legs

• Waxy, mask-like appearance of face

• CREST syndrome (see above)

• Skin darkening or a salt-and-pepper appearance

• Thinning of lips and furrowing around the mouth

• Muscle and joint pain and/or stiffness

• Grating noise with movement of joints

• Weight loss

• Fatigue

• Heartburn

• Gastroparesis (sensation of nausea, fullness, or bloating from retention of food in stomach)

• Cramps and/or diarrhea

• Chronic cough

• Shortness of breath

Muscle and joint pain may also occur along tendons and in muscles in the arms and legs. This can worsen with movement of the ankles, wrists, knees, or elbows. As the disease progresses, muscle loss and weakness may develop along with swelling, warmth, and tenderness around the joints and muscles.

Often, people with diffuse cutaneous SSc experience a grating noise when they try to move inflamed joints, particularly joints at and below the knees.

In the lower GI tract, diffuse cutaneous SSc can sometimes slow movement of food and reduce food absorption.

In both types of systemic sclerosis, lumps of calcinosis may break through the skin and leak a white substance. The open cuts may then become infected.

Rare Symptoms

There are rare subtypes of localized scleroderma that can sometimes develop into more serious conditions:

• **Subcutaneous morphea** affects deeper tissues and can extend deep into muscles.

• **Bullous morphea** causes blister-like bumps or areas of erosion on the region of morphea.

• **Generalized morphea** may also limit joint function due to its larger coverage areas. In rare cases, the larger lesions can merge together, covering the entire body.

• En coup de sabre is a rare form of linear scleroderma that affects the head, especially the forehead. Lesions form depressed grooves that resemble a sword wound or the stroke of a saber. If it's on the scalp, hair loss can occur. In rare cases, en coup de sabre can cause abnormalities in the growth of facial bones and, unlike other forms of localized scleroderma, it can recur many years after going away.

Some people with SSc experience additional symptoms that may or may not seem related to the disease. This can include:

• Trigeminal neuralgia (sudden episodes of severe facial pain)

• Limited eye movement

• Severe fatigue and depression

Diagnosis and Treatment

Diagnosis

There are no specific tests for scleroderma. But, your doctor may suspect you have scleroderma after a physical exam and asking about your symptom history. Part of your physical exam may include:

• Checking for thickened and hardened skin areas (they may use a scoring system, such as the modified Rodnan skin score to help them tell how serious your skin symptoms are)

• Pressing on your tendons and joints to listen and feel for changes that are related to scleroderma

• Looking at your fingernails underneath the microscope for swollen small blood vessels (nailfold capillary test)

• Imaging tests, such as ultrasound and computerized skin scoring, to check how your disease develops over time

• Blood tests to use in antibody testing

• Upper gastrointestinal tests

• Lung function tests, including diffusion capacity

• Heart tests such as an EKG or right heart catheterization

They might also take a small sample of skin (called a biopsy) for a specialist to look at under a microscope.

Scleroderma antibodies

Tests for proteins made by your body called antibodies may also help your doctor diagnose scleroderma and plan your treatment. Some of these antibodies include:

• **Antinuclear antibody (ANA).** Many people who have an autoimmune condition are positive for ANA antibodies, and so are most people with scleroderma.

• **Anti-RNA polymerase 3 (Pol 3).** It is most often positive in people with diffuse scleroderma. People positive for Pol 3 are at a high risk of getting skin thickening and kidney problems.

• Anti-topoisomerase (TOPO or anti-SCL-70). It is mostly positive in people with diffuse scleroderma and in those at high risk of developing interstitial lung disease.

• Anti-centromere antibodies (ACA). These are most often positive in people with limited skin systemic sclerosis and in those who may develop pulmonary artery high blood pressure.

The presence of other antibodies such as anti-fibrillarin, anti-TH/To, anti-U11/U12 RNP, anti-U1 RNP, anti-PM-Sci, and anti-Ku may indicate that you also have another connective tissue disease that overlaps with scleroderma.

Treatment

There is no treatment that can cure or stop the overproduction of collagen that happens in scleroderma. But a variety of treatments can help control symptoms and prevent complications.

Medicines

Because scleroderma can affect so many different parts of the body, the choice of medicine varies depending on the symptoms. Examples include medicines that:

• **Dilate blood vessels.** Blood pressure medicines that dilate blood vessels may help treat Raynaud's phenomenon.

• **Suppress the immune system.** Medicines that suppress the immune system, such as those taken after organ transplants, may help reduce progression of some scleroderma symptoms, such as the thickening of the skin or worsening of lung damage.

• **Reduce digestive symptoms.** Pills to reduce stomach acid can help relieve heartburn. Antibiotics and medicines that help move food through the intestines may help reduce bloating, diarrhea and constipation.

• **Prevent infections**. Recommended vaccinations are important to protect people with scleroderma from infectious diseases. Talk with your healthcare professional about vaccines for influenza, pneumonia, shingles, HPV, COVID-19 and RSV.

• **Relieve pain**. If pain relievers available without a prescription don't help enough, your healthcare professional might suggest prescription medicines to control pain.

Therapies

Physical or occupational therapists can help you improve your strength and mobility and maintain independence with daily tasks. Hand therapy may help prevent hand stiffness, also called contractures.

Surgical and other procedures

Stem cell transplants might be an option for people who have serious symptoms that haven't responded to more-common treatments. If the lungs or kidneys have been badly damaged, organ transplants might be considered.

Outlook for Scleroderma

The outlook for scleroderma can vary widely from person to person. However, many people with scleroderma—particularly those with limited disease—go on to live normal lifespans.

For others, life expectancy can be affected by many factors including how invasive the disease is and whether serious complications have developed.

While there is no cure for scleroderma, there are treatments available that can help relieve symptoms and prevent complications. Treatment is most effective when started early.

Localized scleroderma typically gets better on its own; there will likely come a time when no new lesions form and the existing ones fade. Systemic sclerosis is manageable with treatments to target affected organs. These treatments are continuously improving and can help with symptoms and improve quality of life.

CHAPTER II

SCLERODERMA AND DIET

How Scleroderma Affects Digestion and Nutrient Absorption

Swallowing

Overproduction of collagen due to scleroderma can cause thickening and scarring of tissue. This can result in the slow movement of food through the digestive tract, which is known as dysmotility.

Difficulty in swallowing, or dysphagia, is also common in scleroderma. Another common symptom of scleroderma is dry mouth, or xerostomia. Reduced saliva means that chewed food is less moist, making it harder to swallow.

A speech pathologist may be able to help you to assess and choose the right texture of foods for your specific case.

If you experience any of these issues, these tips may help:

•Eat slowly. Allow more time for eating, due to slower movement of food passing through.

• Chew well. Smaller pieces of food are easier for your body to digest properly.

• Try soft or pureed foods such as mashed potatoes, soup, pureed fruit and casseroles. A slow cooker can be your new best friend!

• Some people may experience problems with dry foods such as bread or biscuits. You can dip them into liquids such as broth or spread some butter to moisten them. • Drink small amounts of fluids frequently and between bites to help the food go down.

• Blending or mincing foods such as meats or vegetables can make them easier to digest. Add seasonings, sauces, or butter to improve the flavour and texture.

The Oesophagus

A common condition that occurs in patients with scleroderma is GORD. GORD, or GastroOesophageal Reflux Disease, can cause irritation in the œsophagus, the pipe that connects the throat to the stomach. This condition is commonly known as 'acid reflux'.

In GORD, the ring of muscle known as the lower oesophageal sphincter becomes damaged or weakened. This allows stomach acid to rise into the œsophagus, causing irritation.

There are liquid supplements available for people with swallowing difficulties. To reduce acid reflux, consider the following:

• Decrease or eliminate the intake of alcohol, fizzy drinks and caffeine, which are common triggers for acid reflux

. • Possible triggers for acid reflux include citrus fruit, tomatoes, tomato products, spicy foods and onions. If you notice your symptoms flaring after consuming these, reduce or eliminate them.

• Fatty and oily foods are another common trigger for reflux. This is because they can relax the lower oesophageal sphincter. Keep your portions of good fats such as olive oil and avocado on the smaller side, avoid high-fat and processed.

• Remain upright for 1 to 2 hours after eating. Avoid eating just before lying down, napping, or going to bed at night.

• Eat smaller, more frequent meals (4- 6 small meals per day).

• Raise the head of your bed by a small amount (~10cm).

• Keep a food diary to establish the foods that cause symptoms. Show this list to your dietitian or nutritionist, so they can help you to adjust your diet.

The Stomach and Intestines

Absorption of nutrients from the gut is compromised in scleroderma due to a number of reasons. Supplementary nutrients may be of use, particularly when there are known digestive issues.

Tips for Acid Reflux Including foods that contain good bacteria or probiotics may be beneficial. Some studies have suggested that specific strains of probiotics may help to relieve digestive symptoms for people with scleroderma.

It's important to start slowly when adding probiotic foods and supplements, as some digestive conditions may be exacerbated with probiotic use. If this occurs, seek professional advice from a qualified health practitioner.

Diarrhea, constipation, bloating and other digestive problems can be unpleasant symptoms of scleroderma. Diarrhea can be caused by medication use, malabsorption of foods, dysmotility and imbalances in gut flora. Foods that have soluble fibre may help with diarrhea.

Soluble fibre sources include bananas, apples, oats and prunes. Avoid highly processed and refined foods, as these may trigger diarrhea. If severe diarrhea or constipation persists, seek professional help.

Constipation can be caused by medication use, malabsorption of foods, dysmotility and imbalances in gut flora. Dehydration and insufficient physical activity can also contribute to constipation.

If you experience constipation, these tips may help:

• Aim for a fluid intake of 1.5 to 2 litres per day, depending on your body weight and needs. This can include broths, smoothies, herbal teas and nutritional supplements. If you have Raynaud's, allow your beverages to come to room temperature, particularly in cold weather.

• Gentle exercise is beneficial for digestion and movement of the bowels. Going for a short walk is a good place to start, but even incidental activity such as light housework or collecting the mail counts.

• Include fibre-rich foods in your diet. Aim for 20 to 35 grams/day. Be sure to add fibre gradually into the diet. You may experience digestive symptoms such as bloating, colicky pain and gas if you increase fibre too quickly. Dietary fibre sources include fruit, vegetables, nuts, seeds, beans, legumes and wholegrains

Managing Specific Scleroderma-related Issues

REFLUX/HEARTBURN: eat small frequent meals to avoid overfilling your stomach; avoid eating within 2-3 hours of bedtime; avoid foods that may aggravate symptoms such as citrus fruits, tomato products, greasy fried foods, coffee, garlic, onions, peppermint, gas-producing foods (such as raw peppers, beans, broccoli, raw onions), spicy foods, carbonated beverages, and alcohol. If you carry extra weight around your midsection, weight loss may also improve symptoms. Use a sleep wedge or elevate head of the bed to elevate your head and torso to prevent regurgitation of stomach contents into airways.

DECREASED GI MOTILITY/CONSTIPATION: exercise, such as walking, helps move food through the digestive tract; eat a high fiber diet with 100% whole grains, fruits and vegetables; take a daily probiotic supplement (such as Align or Culturelle) and/or eat yogurt with active cultures regularly; increase fluid intake.

INFLAMMATION- increase antioxidant intake by choosing deeply colored fruits and vegetables (especially dark green, deep yellow, orange, red, purple, and blue); eat fatty fish, ground flaxseeds, and walnuts for omega-3 fatty acids; eat vitamin E-rich foods such as nuts, seeds, and extra-virgin olive oil; consider taking a 1000 IU Vitamin D3 (cholecalciferol) tablet with your fattiest meal (to allow for better absorption).

FATIGUE- eat small, frequent meals to provide continuous energy and keep blood sugar from dipping low; increase fluid intake; participate in 30-60 minutes of moderate daily exercise such as walking, bike riding, pool exercise, pilates, yoga, or tai chi. Sleep for 7-8 hours each night. If iron levels are low, which is typical of someone with chronic disease, discuss additional iron supplementation with your doctor. If you currently take an iron pill, swallow it down with a juice containing vitamin C to allow for better absorption.

POOR CIRCULATION/RAYNAUD'S- exercise will increase circulation to areas suffering from limited blood flow; if you suffer from finger ulcers, eat animal sources of protein with zinc and iron (such as beef and pork) to accelerate wound healing.

TIGHT, THICKENED SKIN- eat foods rich in vitamin E such as nuts, seeds, wheat germ, and canola, olive, and peanut oils; consider taking 5 mg (5000 mcg) biotin supplement, which may help skin and nails.

Malnutrition for Scleroderma

Even if you try your best to eat a healthy diet, people who suffer from scleroderma are at increased risk of malnutrition. Malnutrition in scleroderma is either caused by inadequate intake of nutritious foods or from poor absorption of nutrients from the gastrointestinal (GI) tract. Someone who eats less due to difficulty chewing, swallowing, and/or preparing his or her own food may suffer from inadequate nutrient intake, thereby causing excessive weight loss and malnutrition. However, someone suffering from extensive GI involvement may be eating enough food, but is unable to absorb the nutrients properly, resulting in specific vitamin or mineral deficiencies, with or without obvious symptoms. Therefore, it is important for everyone with scleroderma to have their nutritional status monitored regularly and to eat healthy foods throughout the day from all the different food groups. Substantial weight loss over a period of 3-6 months can be an indication of inadequate nutrient and calorie intake. Measuring your weight at home at regular intervals can be a simple step towards monitoring your risk of malnutrition.

Symptoms of malnutrition:

• Unexplained 10% or more weight loss over a 3 month period

• Weakness and muscle wasting

• Excessive or new onset fatigue

• Increased susceptibility to infection (weakened immunity)

• delayed wound healing

• Brittle nails and excessive hair loss

• Excessively dry and flaky skin

The symptoms described above are also related to the underlying scleroderma and may be difficult to distinguish from malnutrition. New or worsening symptoms (such as worsening fatigue or excessive weight loss) may indicate malnutrition.

Laboratory tests to diagnose malnutrition:

• Protein malnutrition: blood tests to assess total protein, serum albumin, serum pre-albumin

• Specific vitamin/mineral deficiencies: blood tests to assess serum iron, ferritin, total iron binding capacity, zinc, and B-12

• Small bowel bacterial overgrowth: blood tests to assess serum folate, carotene, and/or vitamin D levels

If you are under-eating due to difficulties chewing or swallowing, try these suggestions:

• blend or juice fresh fruits and vegetables

• make homemade smoothies using fruit, yogurt, 2% milk, Carnation Instant Breakfast and/or whey protein powder

• include soft, moist protein sources at meals and snacks such as cottage cheese, scrambled eggs, yogurt, fish, chicken with gravy, ground meats, macaroni and cheese, and lasagna.

If you have lost an excessive amount of weight, consider the following to help restore weight and nutritional status:

• have your physician rule out small bowel bacterial overgrowth and gastroparesis.

• liberally add sources of healthy fats to your diet by way of olive, canola, and peanut oils; nuts, seeds and nut butters; avocado; fatty fish; and oil-based salad dressings

• make homemade smoothies using fruit, yogurt, 2% milk, 1-2 Tbsp. peanut butter, 1-3 tsp. canola oil, Carnation Instant Breakfast and/or whey protein powder

• consider including a high-protein liquid nutrition supplement (such as Ensure Plus or Boost Plus) between meals 1-3 times per day; if not tolerated, try Boost Breeze, a high protein juice-based alternative

• eat every 2 hours to maximize calorie and nutrient intake

General Diet Recommendations:

• Eat small, frequent meals every 3-4 hours. If you have been experiencing excessive weight loss or can only eat small amounts at one time, consider eating every two hours to maximize nutrient intake.

• Choose fresh, whole, minimally processed foods, without preservatives, artificial ingredients, or hydrogenated oils. If there are "chemical" sounding names in the ingredient list, avoid it. In general, the shorter the ingredient list, the better.

• Add antioxidant rich, anti-inflammatory herbs and spices liberally to foods such as basil, rosemary, oregano, cinnamon, ginger, paprika, cayenne, turmeric, and curry powder.

• Cut down on added sugars. (Natural sugar found in fruit, milk, and yogurt is not a concern unless it causes GI distress.) Check ingredient lists for stealthy terms indicating added sugar such as sucrose, evaporated cane juice, fructose, brown rice syrup, honey, agave nectar, molasses, corn syrup, and maple syrup.

• Consider taking an over the counter multivitamin/mineral supplement containing 15 mg zinc, 10-18 mg iron, vitamins A, D, E, and K, folate, and B-12. If specific nutrient deficiencies have been identified, extra supplementation may be required. Taking a probiotic supplement such as Align or

Culturelle may help restore intestinal function and help with symptoms of bloating and distention.

• Drink fresh, filtered water that has never been exposed to plastic. Use a water filtration system at home and drink only from glass or stainless steel containers. Aim to drink half your body weight in water each day. (i.e. 75 oz. for a 150 lb. person)

CHAPTER III

FOODS AND SUBSTANCES TO INCLUDE AND AVOID

Foods to Include for Improved Immune Function

One of the best ways to stay healthy is by choosing an array of foods to boost your immune system. Eating healthy, antioxidant-rich foods such as fruits and vegetables, whole grains, and lean protein is an important part of maintaining good immune system health to help ward off infection and illness.

White blood cells are a key part of the immune system. These disease-fighters circulate through the body to fight bacteria and viruses, working to slow or stop the illnesses that these germs can cause. So it's important to eat nourishing foods, especially those with protein, vitamin B, and folate, to help make sure your immune system has enough white blood cells to do its job.

While no one food is a silver bullet for optimal immune system function, these have been studied for their potential positive effects, including increasing white blood cells and fighting inflammation (as antioxidants can).

Fish

Omega- fatty acids and other healthy fats help increase the activity of white blood cells. There are a few different kinds of omega s. Oily fish contains docosahexaenoic acid (DHA) and eicosapentaenoic acid (EPA).

Certain nuts and vegetable oils contain alpha-linolenic acid (ALA), which can only be acquired through foods. The body can convert ALA into EPA and DHA, but it's more efficient to consume them in your diet.

Omega-s may also play an important role in the production of compounds that regulate immunity in the body and help protect the body from damage from over-reacting to infections.

Pregnant people and young children should avoid high mercury fish like king mackerel, tilefish, shark, and swordfish.

The best way to get the omega -fatty acids DHA and EPA is by eating fatty fish such as tuna, salmon, and mackerel. You can also get these omega-s through krill oil capsules or algae supplements (which is a vegan source). Other sources of the omega- fatty acid ALA include flax seeds, flax oil, chia seeds, hemp seeds, and walnuts.

Yogurt

When choosing yogurt, go for the style you enjoy the most. It's important to choose a variety that uses live and active cultures. If you opt for plain yogurt and add fruit, spices, and a little of your favorite sweetener, you will have a lower-sugar snack that's also loaded with calcium.

Studies have shown that the live cultures in yogurt can protect the intestinal tract against gastrointestinal illnesses and increase resistance to immune-related diseases such as infection and even cancer.

The beneficial live cultures in yogurt, such as lactobacillus acidophilus, may help prevent colds and other infections or shorten their duration, although more research is needed. Yogurt can also be a good source of protein, which the body uses to make white blood cells.

Poultry and Lean Meats

Foods high in protein, such as lean meats and poultry, are high in zinc—a mineral that increases white blood cells and T-cells, which fight infection. Other great sources of zinc are oysters, nuts, fortified cereal, and beans.

Brightly-Colored Vegetables

Carotenoids such as beta-carotene are important antioxidants that aid in immune system function. Carotenoids are present in bright yellow, orange, and red fruits and vegetables, although they can also be found in fruits and veggies that are mostly green.

It's important to get a variety of fruits and vegetables of different colors because various types of carotenoids are thought to work together to strengthen the body's immune system.

Nuts

These protein-packed powerhouses of vitamins and minerals are rich in antioxidants such as vitamin E, omega- fatty acids, and zinc.

Studies have shown a link between eating nuts and health benefits such as a lower risk of chronic disease.

Berries

Berries are rich in vitamin C and bioflavonoids, phytochemicals found in fruits and vegetables that may work as antioxidants and prevent injury to cells.

One cup of strawberries contains as much as milligrams of vitamin C, which is nearly as much as a cup of orange juice. Dark berries such as blueberries are especially high in bioflavonoids. For an optimal immune system boosting effect, eat a bowl of mixed berries, or vary which berries you choose from day to day, rather than eating just one type.

Garlic

Most of the clinical studies done on garlic's potential antibacterial and antiviral properties use concentrated extracts. However, historically, cloves of garlic have been used in food for an assortment of health-related reasons. If you enjoy garlic, it doesn't hurt to include it in your meals and it is possible that some of the health benefits seen from the extracts also translate to culinary uses.

Mushrooms

Mushrooms may be a potent weapon in warding off colds, flu, and other infections. Studies on fresh mushrooms, dried mushrooms, and extracts have shown that mushrooms such as shiitake, maitake, and reishi have antiviral, antibacterial, and anti-tumor effects.

Chocolate

Here's some happy news for chocolate lovers everywhere: Some studies indicate that cocoa and extracts of cocoa might positively affect various aspects of the immune system as well as act as a powerful antioxidant. As long as you keep the sugar and fat to a minimum, unsweetened cocoa and cocoa powder may play a role in immune system health.

The studies on cocoa are often done on extracts, although they may extrapolate the amount of extract used to a correlating amount of cocoa.

Recent studies have also looked at cocoa as a whole and even dark chocolate.

Studies have shown that regular consumption of cocoa/extracts may reduce heart disease risk, help raise good cholesterol, and possibly reverse blood vessel damage in people with diabetes.

Persimmons

Demonstrating good timing, these delicious fruits make their appearance right around cold and flu season. Persimmons are high in vitamins A and C, which are important for immune system function.

Just one medium persimmon has about half of the recommended daily allowance of vitamin A, which has been shown to play a key role in the regulation of immune cells.

• Other sources of vitamin A: Pumpkins, sweet potatoes, butternut squash, spinach

• Other sources of vitamin C: Strawberries, papaya, kiwi, cantaloupe, oranges

Foods to Avoid or Limit to Reduce Inflammation

These include foods with few nutrients that are often ultra-processed, fried, and high in added sugar, salt, or saturated fat. Think potato chips instead of potatoes.

Examples of inflammatory foods include:

Sweets, cakes, cookies, and soda. They aren't dense in nutrients and they're easy to overeat. This can lead to weight gain, high blood sugar, and high cholesterol (all related to inflammation). Sugar causes your body to release inflammatory messengers called cytokines. It's best to avoid or limit food and drinks with added sugars, including agave and honey, if possible.

Red and processed meat. Red meat comes from cows, pigs, sheep, and goats. It includes things like burgers and steaks. Along with processed meat like bacon, hot dogs, and sausage, these meats have a lot of pro-inflammatory saturated fat.

Butter, whole milk, and cheese. These foods tend to be high in saturated fat, unlike low-fat dairy products.

Fried foods. Some vegetable oils like corn oil, safflower oil, and soybean oil are high in omega-6 fatty acids. You need some omega-6s, but if you get too much, you throw off the balance between omega-6s and omega-3s in your body and end up with more inflammation.

Anything with trans fats. These often show up on packaged food labels as "partially hydrogenated oils." A diet high in trans fats can raise LDL cholesterol and your chances of heart disease, stroke, and type 2 diabetes.

Gluten-containing foods like wheat, rye, and barley. They aren't harmful to everyone. But people who have celiac disease have an immune reaction when they eat gluten, and they have to avoid this protein completely. Gluten may also promote inflammation in folks with a non-celiac gluten or wheat sensitivity.

Alcohol. Light or moderate drinking may lower certain types of inflammation. But if you drink more than a glass of wine or beer a day, the opposite may happen. Ask your doctor how much alcohol, if any, is safe for you.

Key Nutrients for Scleroderma Patients

Many people living with scleroderma experience symptoms that can lead to a poor appetite and weight loss. Because of this, it is really important to choose a balanced diet and maintain weight within a healthy range. Doing so may help you to avoid the risk of developing heart, lung and kidney problems.

Some important elements to include in your diet include all of the following:

Calcium is important for healthy bones. Milk and dairy products are good sources of calcium. Other sources of calcium include; fish, dark green vegetables, pulses, seeds, nuts and fortified cereals. If you are taking steroids your body's requirements for calcium will be increased.

Vitamin D is obtained from sunlight and is needed to help absorb and utilise calcium. Vitamin D can also be found in certain fortified foods such as eggs, fat spreads (butter and margarine) and cereals.

Iron reduces the risk of anaemia with an adequate intake. It can be found in red meat, poultry, fish, eggs and dark green leafy vegetables. Drinking a small amount of orange juice can help absorb iron due to the vitamin C content. Tea can reduce iron absorption, so should be avoided at meal times.

Omega 3 fats can help to protect against many diseases including heart disease, and they can reduce inflammation in arthritis. They are also known to have a positive effect on mood. Sources of omega-3 include oily fish (such as sardines, mackerel, pilchards, salmon and fresh tuna), rapeseed oil and walnuts, as well as fortified eggs and margarines.

The following fruits, vegetables and spices are believed to be particularly helpful for some people in managing scleroderma:

• **Ginger** is found by many people to be a powerful anti-oxidant that has anti-inflammatory properties. Ginger may inhibit pain-producing prostaglandins

• **Turmeric** contains curcumin, which is also believed to have anti-inflammatory and pain-relieving properties

• **Tart red cherries** are found by some people to relieve pain and inflammation, if about 20 per day are eaten

• **Fresh pineapple** contains an enzyme called bromelain that is believed to be a powerful anti-inflammatory; it is also thought to help in the digestion of protein-rich foods. Two to three slices a day may help with recovery from surgery and enhance circulation

• The following foods groups, if tolerated, each offer their own nutritional benefits, which may potentially help with managing a long-term health condition such as scleroderma:

• **Fruits and vegetables** help to reduce pain and inflammation. They are also a good source of fibre, and help to regulate blood pressure and blood fats.

 Aim for five portions of fruit and vegetable portions per day – one portion = 80g. Be aware that if you have heartburn and reflux, you might be better off avoiding acidic citrus fruits.

• **Starchy foods** are a good source of energy and the main source of a range of nutrients in our diet. As well as starch, they contain fibre, calcium, iron and B vitamins.

• **Beta-glucan,** which is believed to be helpful in managing scleroderma, is found in cereal grains like barley, oats, rye and wheat. Include at least two portions at every meal – one portion = one slice of bread (40g), two to three heaped tablespoons of rice and pasta, three to four heaped tablespoons of breakfast cereal, or two medium-sized boiled potatoes.

• **Milk and dairy products** are a good source of protein and calcium. Aim for two to three portions of dairy foods per day – one portion = 30g of cheese, one small pot of yoghurt (150ml), or 200ml of milk.

• **Protein-rich foods** help the body to grow and repair, so they are particularly important when you are recovering from surgery or ulcers. Aim for two to three portions of protein per day, including one to two portions of oily fish per week. One portion = 80g of cooked meat, poultry or oily fish, 120g of white fish, three tablespoons of baked beans, red kidney beans, chick peas or lentils, or one to two eggs.

• **Foods high in fat and sugar** can have negative effects on health, so need to be kept to moderate amounts.

CHAPTER IV

NOURISHING BREAKFAST RECIPES FOR SCLERODERMA

Low FODMAP Shakshuka

INGREDIENTS

• 1 tablespoon garlic-infused olive oil

• ½ cup finely chopped leek leaves (dark green parts only)

• 1 cup diced red bell pepper (about 1 pepper)

• 2 cups Fody Foods Low FODMAP Arrabbiata Sauce (about 1 jar)

• 1 tablespoon ground cumin

• 4 large eggs

• 2 cups cooked brown (or white) rice

Optional Garnishes

• 2 tablespoons chopped fresh parsley

• ¼ cup crumbled feta cheese

INSTRUCTIONS

1. Heat a large nonstick skillet over medium-high heat. Once hot, add the olive oil, leek leaves (dark green parts only), and red bell pepper. Saute, stirring occasionally, until the bell pepper pieces are fork-tender and the leek leaves are bright green, soft, and fragrant.

2. Reduce heat to medium. Stir in the low FODMAP arrabbiata and ground cumin. Heat until the sauce is just about to boil.

3. Mentally divide the skillet into quarters. In one quarter, create a well with a spatula. Carefully crack an egg into the well. To help prevent shell fragments, you may want to crack the egg into a small bowl before pouring it into the well. Repeat with the remaining eggs.

4. Cover the skillet and cook until the eggs are cooked to your preference. I usually cook until the egg whites have turned an opaque white, and the yolks are still soft with just a little jiggle when I shake the skillet. If you prefer more fully-cooked yolks, continue to cook until there is little to no jiggle. The eggs will continue to cook a little after removing from heat.

5. Serve warm over cooked rice topped with optional fresh parsley and feta cheese.

Dairy Free French Toast

Ingredients

• 2 large organic eggs

• 1 tablespoon unsweetened almond milk

• 1/4 tsp cinnamon

• 1/8 tsp vanilla extract

• 1 tablespoon olive oil or vegan butter

• 4 slices gluten-free bread (any brand, I love Little Northern Bakehouse or Udi's)

OPTIONAL TOPPINGS:

• Pure Maple Syrup

• Sliced Banana

• Fresh Berries

• Coconut Yogurt

Instructions

1. In a bowl whisk together the eggs, almond milk, cinnamon, and vanilla until smooth.

2. Transfer egg mixture to a wide shallow bowl.

3. Heat a large non-stick pan or skillet over medium-high heat and add oil or butter.

4. Dredge 1 slice of bread into the egg mixture and flip back and forth to make sure each side is coated with the egg mixture and is slightly soaking into the bread.

5. Add 1-2 soaked bread slices to the pan and cook for 2 minutes on each side until just golden brown.

6. Repeat the process for all slices of bread (you should use up all of the egg mixture with the 4 slices of bread).

7. Stack the french toast slices, layering with sliced banana, top with a dollop of vegan butter and berries, and then drizzle with pure maple syrup.

8. Enjoy!

Creamy Blueberry Avocado Smoothie

Ingredients

• 3/4 cup fresh or frozen blueberries

• 1/4 of an avocado (green flesh only)

• 1/2 banana, frozen*

• 1/2 tsp cinnamon

• 2 large pitted dates

• 3/4 cup unsweetened vanilla almond milk

• 1 scoop vanilla plant protein powder of your choice (1/4 cup) or 2 heaping tablespoons unflavoured collagen peptides (not vegan)

Instructions

1. Add all Ingredients to a high-speed blender or Vitamix and blend until completely smooth.

2. Enjoy immediately.

Low FODMAP Quinoa Porridge with Berries and Cinnamon

Ingredients

Quinoa Porridge with Berries

85 quinoa*

1   neutral oil (rice bran, canola, sunflower)

250 water

187.5 low FODMAP milk*

0.25 ground cinnamon*

4 pure maple syrup*

10 raspberries (fresh or frozen)

20 blueberries (fresh or frozen)

Directions

1. Measure out the quinoa. Using a fine mesh sieve rinse it under cold running water for two minutes. Transfer it to a medium sized saucepan and add a drizzle of neutral oil. Toast the quinoa over medium heat for 1 to 2 minutes until the water has

evaporated and the quinoa is lightly toasted. Add the water. Bring the quinoa to a rolling boil and then turn down the element to the lowest heat setting. Cover with a pot lid and allow to cook for 12 to 15 minutes. The quinoa should be quite fluffy. Drain off any excess water if needed and return to pan.

2. Then add the low FODMAP milk, cinnamon, and maple syrup. If all the low FODMAP milk disappears you can add a little bit more. Then allow the porridge to simmer for about 5 minutes or until heated through. If you are using frozen berries and want them heated then add them to the mixture.

3. Serve the hot quinoa porridge into bowls and divide the raspberries and blueberries equally between them.

Caramelised Banana with Low FODMAP Porridge

Ingredients

Caramelised Banana with Porridge

1/2 cup   rice flakes or rolled oats*

125 ml (1/2 cup)   low FODMAP milk (double the milk if using oats)*

80 g (1 small)   bananas (firm - no brown spots) (sliced)*

2 tsp   neutral oil (rice bran, canola, sunflower)

2 tsp   pure maple syrup*

1/4 tsp   vanilla extract

1/16 tsp   ground cinnamon (about a pinch)*

Directions

1. Cook your porridge (rice porridge or oats) according to packet Directions using the low FODMAP milk.

2. Heat a small saucepan over the medium heat. Add the neutral oil, maple syrup, a sprinkle of cinnamon and a dash of vanilla extract. Allow to bubble for a minute. Then add the sliced banana. Cook for 2 to 3 minutes, until the banana is plump and golden.

3. Top the cooked porridge with the caramelised banana.

Low FODMAP Salmon & Spinach Omelette with Cherry Tomatoes

Ingredients

Salmon & Spinach Omelette

6   large egg

1.5   low FODMAP milk*

0.125   paprika*

1   salt & pepper

2   neutral oil (rice bran, canola, sunflower)

210   plain pink salmon (canned)*

2   sesame oil

60   spinach (washed & finely shredded)

2   fresh parsley (finely chopped)

6   cherry tomato

Directions

1. Mix the eggs together with the low FODMAP milk until well combined. Then season with salt and pepper.

2. Heat a medium sized non-stick fry pan over medium-low heat, add a little bit of neutral oil and pour the egg mixture in. Alternatively you can cook smaller omelettes in a small non-stick fry pan, but you will need to cook them one after another which is a bit more time consuming. Sprinkle paprika over the top of the omelette mixture and cook until firm. Turn down the heat to medium low. If the top of the omelette isn't cooked after eight minutes, flip the omelette and cook for a further minute or place it in the oven under high grill. Make sure you keep an eye on the pan while the omelette cooks, and turn down the heat if the omelette looks like it might burn.

3. While the omelette cooks prepare the salmon and spinach. Drain the salmon and then remove it from the tin. Place the salmon in a small bowl and mix through the sesame oil, parsley and some salt and pepper. Heat a large non-stick fry pan over medium heat, add the salmon mixture and heat through. Then add the washed and shredded spinach and cook until the spinach wilts.

4. Serve the salmon and spinach mixture on the omelette and top with halved cherry tomatoes and a few grinds of black pepper.

Blueberry Lime Coconut Smoothie

Ingredients

- 1/2 cup fresh or frozen blueberries

- 2 tablespoons flaked coconut

• 2 tablespoons fresh lime juice

• 4 ounces plain nonfat lactose free yogurt (I used Green Valley)

• 1 teaspoon chia seeds

• 2 tablespoons water

• Ice if using fresh blueberries (about 6 cubes or more depending on desired thickness)

Instructions

1. Add Ingredients to blender and blend away until frothy.

Crumpets

Ingredients

• 2½ tsp dried yeast

• 240ml warm milk

• 2 tbsp unsalted butter, melted

• 2tsp sea salt

• 2tsp caster sugar

• 470g plain flour

• ½ tsp baking powder dissolved in 60ml warm water

• vegetable oil, to grease

• butter or cheese, to serve

Instructions

• STEP 1

Stir together the yeast and 240ml warm water in a bowl and leave to stand for 5-10 mins. Add the warm milk, butter, salt and sugar, then tip in the flour and stir until smooth. Leave to stand for 30 mins.

• STEP 2

Dissolve the baking powder in a little water, then leave to rise for 20-30 mins.

• STEP 3

Oil a heavy-based frying pan with a little vegetable oil and heat over medium-low heat. Lightly oil four 9cm crumpet rings. Spoon batter into the rings so it comes halfway up the sides. Reduce heat to low, cover with a lid, or an upturned deep frying pan to give the crumpets space to rise. Cook until the tops look dry, about 10-12 mins.

• STEP 4

Flip them over and cook for 5 mins until golden and firm. Repeat with the remaining batter. Serve toasted with butter or topped with cheese, melted under the grill.

Cinnamon roll pancakes

Ingredients

• 145g self-raising flour

• 1 tsp baking powder

• 1 tbsp golden caster sugar

• 1 tsp cinnamon

• 2 eggs

• 40g butter, melted

• 140ml milk

• 3 tbsp light brown soft sugar

- 1 tbsp maple syrup, plus extra to serve (optional)

- 1 tbsp vegetable oil

- 6 tbsp toffee or caramel yogurt, to serve (optional)

Instructions

- STEP 1

Weigh the flour in a large jug or bowl. Add the baking powder, caster sugar, ½ tsp cinnamon and a generous pinch of salt. Whisk to combine. Crack in the eggs, add ½ the butter and all the milk, then whisk to a smooth batter. Will keep in the fridge overnight.

- STEP 2

Stir the rest of the cinnamon, the light brown sugar and the maple syrup into the remaining melted butter. Add 3 tbsp of the pancake mixture and mix.

Transfer to a squeezy bottle fitted with a small nozzle or a piping bag.

• STEP 3

When you're ready to cook, pour a little oil in your largest frying pan, and wipe out any excess with some kitchen paper. Keeping the pan over a low-medium heat, spoon 2-3 tbsp mounds into the pan for each pancake, leaving space for them to expand as they cook. You should get three or four in at a time. Use the cinnamon mixture in your bottle or piping bag to pipe swirls on top of each pancake. When the pancakes start to set around the edges and you see bubbles appear on top, carefully flip and cook for another 2-3 mins until golden and cooked through. Keep warm in a low oven while you continue cooking the rest of the batter.

• STEP 4

Serve the pancakes with yogurt and extra maple syrup, if you like.

Brown loaf

Ingredients

• 400g malted grain brown bread flour, or wholemeal or granary bread flour

• 100g strong white bread flour

• 7g sachet easy-bake dried yeast (or 2 tsp Quick dried yeast)

• 1½ tsp salt

• 1 tbsp soft butter

• 4 tbsp mixed seed (optional), such as linseed, pumpkin, sesame and sunflower, plus extra for sprinkling

Instructions

- STEP 1

Mix your choice of brown flour with the white, the yeast and salt in a large mixing bowl. Put in the butter and rub it into the flour. Stir in the seeds if using. Make a dip in the centre of the flour and pour in almost 300ml hand warm (cool rather than hot) water, with a round-bladed knife. Then mix in enough of the remaining water and a bit more if needed, to gather up any dry bits in the bottom of the bowl and until the mixture comes together as a soft, not too sticky, dough. Gather it into a ball with your hands.

- STEP 2

Put the dough on to a very lightly floured surface and knead for 8-10 mins until it feels smooth and elastic, only adding the minimum of extra flour if necessary to prevent the dough sticking. Place the ball of dough on a lightly floured work surface. Cover with an upturned, clean, large glass bowl and leave for 45 mins-1 hr or until doubled in size and feels light and springy. Timing will depend on the warmth of the room.

• STEP 3

Knock back the dough by lightly kneading just 3-4 times. You only want to knock out any large air bubbles, so too much handling now will lose the dough's lightness. Shape into a ball. Cover with the glass bowl and leave for 15 mins.

• STEP 4

Now shape to make a tin loaf Grease a 1.2-litre capacity loaf tin (about 23 x 13 x 5.5cm) and line the base with baking parchment. Using your knuckles, flatten the dough into a rectangle about 25 x 19cm.

Fold both shorter ends into the centre like an envelope, make a ¼ turn, then flatten again into the same size and roll up very tightly, starting from one of the short ends. Roll the top of the dough in extra seeds and place in the tin with the join underneath, pressing the seeds gently into the dough. Cover with a clean tea towel. Leave for 40-45 mins, or until risen about 5cm above the top of the tin.

• STEP 5

Put a roasting tin in the bottom of the oven 20 mins before ready to bake and heat oven to 230C/210C fan/gas 8. Put the risen bread in the oven, carefully pour about 250ml cold water into the roasting tin (this will hiss and create a burst of steam to give you a crisp crust), then lower the heat to 220C/200C fan/gas 7. Bake for about 30 mins or until golden, covering with foil for the last 5 mins if starting to brown too quickly. Leave in the tin for 2-3 mins, then remove and cool on a wire rack. If you tap the underneath of the baked loaf if should be firm and sound hollow.

Chocolate chip pancakes

Ingredients

• 300g self-raising flour

• 1 tsp baking powder

• 3 tbsp caster sugar

• 2 medium eggs

• 300ml whole milk

• 150g milk chocolate chips

• butter, for frying

• whipped cream or ice cream, to serve (optional)

Instructions

- STEP 1

Sieve the flour, baking powder and ¼ tsp salt into a large mixing bowl. Add the caster sugar and stir until well combined.

- STEP 2

Whisk the eggs and milk together in a jug. Make a well in the centre of the dry Ingredients and pour in the wet Ingredients. Use a whisk to combine everything and create a smooth batter. Fold through most of the chocolate chips.

- STEP 3

Heat a small knob of butter in a large non-stick frying pan over a medium heat, swirling it round to coat the pan. Add 2-3 tbsp of the batter to the pan and cook for 1-2 mins, or until bubbles begin to rise to the surface. Flip the pancake over and cook for 2 mins on the other side for the same amount of time, or until golden brown and puffed up. Repeat with the remaining batter, keeping the pancakes warm in a low oven.

• STEP 4

Stack the pancakes on plates and top with any leftover chocolate chips and a dollop of whipped cream or ice cream, if you like.

Creamy yogurt porridge with apple & raisin compote

Ingredients

For the compote

• 2 apples, peeled and thickly sliced

- 25g raisin

- 150ml orange juice

- small handful of sunflower seeds

For the porridge

- 6 tbsp (50g) porridge oat

- 300g pot 0% fat probiotic plain yogurt

Instructions

- STEP 1

For the apple topping: Poach apples in a covered pan with raisins and orange juice for 8-10 mins until the apple is tender. Mash a little of the apple to thicken the juice. Can be made ahead and chilled for up to 1 week. Serve warm or cold on the porridge with sunflower seeds.

• STEP 2

For the porridge: Tip 400ml water into a small non-stick pan and stir in porridge oats. Cook over a low heat until bubbling and thickened. (To make in a microwave, use a deep container to prevent spillage as the mixture will rise up as it cooks, and cook for 3 mins on High.) Stir in yogurt – or swirl in half and top with the rest.

Kedgeree

Ingredients

• 50g butter

• 1 medium onion, finely chopped

• 3 cardamom pods split open

• ¼ tsp turmeric

- 1 small cinnamon stick

- 2 fresh bay leaves or 1 dried

- 450g basmati rice

- 1 litre/1¾ pints chicken stock or fish stock, ideally fresh

- 750g un-dyed smoked haddock fillet

- 3 eggs

- 3 tbsp chopped fresh parsley

- 1 lemon, cut into wedges, to garnish

Instructions

- STEP 1

Melt 50g butter in a large saucepan (about 20cm across), add 1 finely chopped medium onion and cook gently over a medium heat for 5 minutes, until softened but not browned.

• STEP 2

Stir in 3 split cardamom pods, ¼ tsp turmeric, 1 small cinnamon stick and 2 bay leaves, then cook for 1 minute.

• STEP 3

Tip in 450g basmati rice and stir until it is all well coated in the spicy butter.

• STEP 4

Pour in 1 litre chicken or fish stock, add ½ teaspoon salt and bring to the boil, stir once to release any rice from the bottom of the pan. Cover with a close-fitting lid, reduce the heat to low and leave to cook very gently for 12 minutes.

• STEP 5

Meanwhile, bring some water to the boil in a large shallow pan. Add 750g un-dyed smoked haddock fillet and simmer for 4 minutes, until the fish is just cooked. Lift it out onto a plate and leave until cool enough to handle.

• STEP 6

Hard-boil 3 eggs for 8 minutes.

• STEP 7

Flake the fish, discarding any skin and bones. Drain the eggs, cool slightly, then peel and chop.

• STEP 8

Uncover the rice and remove the bay leaves, cinnamon stick and cardamom pods if you wish to. Gently fork in the fish and the chopped eggs, cover again and return to the heat for 2-3 minutes, or until the fish has heated through.

• STEP 9

Gently stir in almost all the 3 tbsp chopped fresh parsley, and season with a little salt and black pepper to taste. Serve scattered with the remaining parsley and garnished with 1 lemon, cut into wedges.

Vegan tomato & mushroom pancakes

Ingredients

• 140g white self-raising flour

• 1 tsp soya flour

• 400ml soya milk

• vegetable oil, for frying

For the topping

• 2 tbsp vegetable oil

• 250g button mushrooms

• 250g cherry tomatoes, halved

• 2 tbsp soya cream or soya milk

• large handful pine nuts

• snipped chives, to serve

Instructions

• STEP 1

Sift the flours and a pinch of salt into a blender. Add
the soya milk and blend to make a smooth batter.

• STEP 2

Heat a little oil in a medium non-stick frying pan until very hot. Pour about 3 tbsp of the batter into the pan and cook over a medium heat until bubbles appear on the surface of the pancake. Flip the pancake over with a palette knife and cook the other side until golden brown. Repeat with the remaining batter, keeping the cooked pancakes warm as you go. You will make about 8.

• STEP 3

For the topping, heat the oil in a frying pan. Cook the mushrooms until tender, add the tomatoes and cook for a couple of mins. Pour in the soya cream or milk and pine nuts, then gently cook until combined. Divide the pancakes between 2 plates, then spoon over the tomatoes and mushrooms. Scatter with chives.

CHAPTER VI

NOURISHING LUNCH RECIPES FOR SCLERODERMA

Roasted new potato, kale & feta salad with avocado

Ingredients

• 200g Jersey Royal potatoes, halved

• 2 garlic cloves

• 2 tbsp cold-pressed rapeseed oil

• 1 lemon, juiced

• 1 banana shallot, chopped

• 200g bag kale

• 1 small ripe avocado, flesh scooped out

• ½ tsp Dijon mustard

• 25g feta (or vegetarian alternative), crumbled

• ½-1 tsp chilli flakes

• 1 tbsp pumpkin seeds, toasted

Directions

• STEP 1

Heat oven to 200C/180C fan/gas 6. Boil the potatoes for 10 mins until mostly tender, drain and leave to steam dry. Toss the potatoes in a large roasting tin with the garlic, drizzle over 1 tbsp oil and season. Roast for 20 mins.

• STEP 2

While the potatoes are roasting, squeeze half the lemon juice over the shallot and half of the kale, season, then massage gently to encourage the kale to soften.

• STEP 3

Remove the garlic cloves from the oven. Put the rest of the kale on top of the potatoes, drizzle over a little oil, season and return to the oven for 5 mins until crisp.

• STEP 4

Meanwhile, blitz the garlic, avocado, mustard, remaining oil and lemon juice together, add enough water to create a smooth dressing and season to taste. Mix the potatoes and cooked kale into the raw kale salad and tip onto a platter. Drizzle over the dressing, then top with the feta, chilli flakes and pumpkin seeds.

Leek, kale & potato soup topped with shoestring fries

Ingredients

• 4 large potatoes (around 500g), 3 peeled and cubed, 1 left whole with skin on

• 1 tbsp cold pressed rapeseed oil

• 15g butter

• 5 leeks (around 500g), washed and sliced into half moons

• 2 garlic cloves, sliced

• 1 ½l vegetable stock (we used Bouillon)

• 200g kale

• 2 tbsp half-fat crème fraîche

Directions

Directions

• STEP 1

Heat oven to 220C/200C fan/ gas 7 and line a baking tray with parchment. Cut the whole potato into matchsticks using a julienne peeler, or shave thin slices using a vegetable peeler, then cut into matchsticks. Pat dry using kitchen paper, then toss with the oil and some seasoning. Spread out on the tray and roast for 15-18 mins.

• STEP 2

Melt the butter in a large saucepan. Add the leeks, chopped potatoes and a pinch of salt, then cook gently for 10 mins until the leeks have softened. Stir in the garlic and cook for 1 min more, then pour in the stock. Simmer for 10-12 mins until the potatoes are soft, then add the kale and cook for 2-3 mins to wilt.

• STEP 3

Stir in the crème fraîche, then blitz with a hand blender and season to taste. Divide the soup between bowls and top with the shoestring fries.

Kale & goat's cheese frittata

Ingredients

• 1 tbsp olive oil

• 2 red onions, thinly sliced

• 200g chopped curly kale

• 2 tbsp balsamic vinegar

• 8 large eggs, lightly beaten with a little seasoning

• 100g firm goat's cheese, broken into chunks

Directions

• STEP 1

Heat oven to 190C/170C fan/gas 5. Heat the oil in a 25cm ovenproof frying pan. Add the onions and cook for 10-15 mins until soft and caramelised. Add the kale and 1 tbsp water, and cook for 5 mins until the kale has wilted. Pour in the balsamic vinegar and bubble for 1 min, then add the eggs. Give everything a quick stir, then leave undisturbed to cook over a low-medium heat for 5 mins until the egg is nearly set and the frittata is turning golden brown on the bottom.

• STEP 2

Scatter the goat's cheese over the top of the frittata. Cook in the oven for 10-15 mins until the cheese is bubbling and the frittata is set in the centre.

Griddled squid, lentil, roast pepper & preserved lemon with tahini

Ingredients

- 3 large red peppers, halved and deseeded

- 4 tbsp extra virgin olive oil, plus a little extra for roasting and frying

- ½ small onion, finely chopped

- 1 celery stick, diced

- 225g puy lentils

- 1 lemon, juiced

- ½ small bunch parsley, chopped

- 600g cleaned and prepared squid

• 2 green and 2 red chillies, halved, deseeded and finely sliced

• 2 garlic cloves, finely sliced

• 1 preserved lemon, flesh removed and discarded, rind very finely sliced

For the tahini dressing

• 4 tbsp tahini

• 2 tbsp Greek yogurt

• 2 tbsp extra virgin olive oil

• 2 garlic cloves, crushed

• ½ lemon, juiced

• ½ small bunch coriander, finely chopped

Directions

• STEP 1

Heat the oven to 200C/180C fan/ gas 6. Put the peppers on a baking tray and brush with some olive oil. Roast for 25-30 mins, until soft and blistered. Leave to cool slightly.

• STEP 2

To make the dressing, combine everything together until it is the consistency of double cream. If it's too thick, add a little water and adjust the seasoning to taste. Set aside. Slice the peppers into strips.

• STEP 3

Heat a little olive oil in a medium pan and fry the onion and celery for 10 mins until soft but not coloured. Tip in the lentils and cover with water. Bring to the boil, then reduce the heat and simmer for 15 mins, or until the lentils are tender, topping up the water if needed.

• STEP 4

Drain the lentils, then spoon into a serving bowl. Season well, then stir in 1 tbsp olive oil, half the lemon juice and the parsley. Leave to cool a bit, then add the peppers.

• STEP 5

Cut the 'wings' from the squid and put them aside with the tentacles. Slice the bodies down one side so they open out, then clean the inside by running a knife blade firmly over the flesh. Score the flesh on the inside, ensuring you don't cut all the way through. Pat dry with kitchen paper, then transfer to a bowl with just enough olive oil to moisten the pieces (about 2 tbsp). Heat a griddle pan until very hot.

• STEP 6

Season the squid and griddle in batches for 20-30 seconds on each side until just golden. Cut into bite-sized pieces, then toss through the lentil salad and drizzle over the remaining lemon juice.

• STEP 7

In a small frying pan, heat 1 tbsp oil and fry the chillies and garlic until golden. Pour over the squid, then toss through the preserved lemon. Serve with the dressing spooned over or on the side.

Sweet & sour radicchio with toasted crumbs & herby lentils

Ingredients

• 5 tbsp extra virgin olive oil or rapeseed oil, plus extra for drizzling

• 1 small red onion, finely chopped

- 15g flat-leaf parsley, leaves picked and finely chopped, stalks finely chopped

- 2 garlic cloves, crushed

- 400g can black or green lentils, drained

- 15g mint, leaves picked and finely chopped

- 3 tbsp sherry or red wine vinegar

- 100g sourdough or focaccia, pulsed to fine crumbs in a food processor

- 1 radicchio (about 500g), quartered, cored and leaves separated

Directions

- STEP 1

Heat 1 tbsp of the oil in a medium saucepan over a medium heat and fry the onion with a pinch of sea salt flakes for 4-5 mins until starting to soften but not colour.

• STEP 2

Add the parsley stalks and half the garlic to the onions, then tip in the lentils and 300ml water. Bring to a simmer and cook for 5 mins, shuffling the pan occasionally – when ready, the lentils should be loose and a little brothy (but not soupy). Add two-thirds of the chopped parsley leaves, two-thirds of the mint, 1 tbsp more oil and 2 tsp of the vinegar. Simmer for 2 mins, then reduce the heat to low just to keep warm.

• STEP 3

Meanwhile, heat 2 tbsp of the oil in a large frying pan over a medium- high heat. After 45 seconds or so, fry the breadcrumbs for 3-4 mins, tossing to coat and stirring occasionally until golden. Reduce the heat to low, stir in the remaining garlic and parsley leaves, cook for 1 min, then transfer to a bowl. Wipe the pan clean with kitchen paper.

• STEP 4

Heat another 1 tbsp oil in the pan over a medium-high heat and cook the radicchio leaves for 1 min, turning often using tongs until they become glossy and slightly wilted (you may need to do this in batches at first, then put all the leaves in the pan once they've all wilted). Make a gap in the middle using a spoon and add the rest of the vinegar along with 1 tbsp water. Turn off the heat and quickly stir the leaves around the pan to wilt further in the steam. Season with sea salt and the remaining mint.

• STEP 5

Divide the lentils between two shallow bowls or plates. Drizzle with a little more oil, top with the leaves and any pan juices, and scatter over the crumbs to serve.

Veggie shepherd's pie with sweet potato mash

Ingredients

• 1 tbsp olive oil

• 1 large onion, halved and sliced

• 2 large carrots (500g/1lb 2oz in total), cut into sugar-cube size pieces

• 2 tbsp thyme chopped

• 200ml red wine

• 400g can chopped tomatoes

• 2 vegetable stock cubes

• 410g can green lentils

• 950g sweet potatoes, peeled and cut into chunks

• 25g butter

• 85g vegetarian mature cheddar, grated

Directions

• STEP 1

Heat 1 tbsp olive oil in a frying pan, then fry 1 halved and sliced large onion until golden.

• STEP 2

Add 2 large carrots, cut into sugar-cube size pieces and most of the 2 tbsp chopped thyme, reserving a sprinkling for later.

• STEP 3

Pour in 200ml red wine, 150ml water and a 400g chopped tomatoes, then crumble in 2 vegetable stock cubes and simmer for 10 mins.

• STEP 4

Tip in a 410g can green lentils, including the juice, then cover and simmer for another 10 mins until the carrots still have a bit of bite and the lentils are pulpy.

• STEP 5

Meanwhile, boil 950g sweet potatoes, cut into chunks, for 15 mins until tender, drain well, then mash with 25g butter and season to taste.

• STEP 6

Pile the lentil mixture into a pie dish, spoon the mash on top, then sprinkle over 85g grated vegetarian mature cheddar and the remaining thyme. The pie can now be covered and chilled for 2 days, or frozen for up to a month.

• STEP 7

Heat oven to 190C/170C fan/gas 5. Cook for 20 mins if cooking straightaway, or for 40 mins from chilled, until golden and hot all the way through. Serve with broccoli.

Lentil & red pepper salad with a soft egg

Ingredients

• 2 eggs

• 400g can green lentils, rinsed and drained

• 1 small red onion, thinly sliced

• 1 red pepper, finely chopped

- 1 tbsp balsamic vinegar

- handful rocket leaves

- 1 tbsp olive oil

Directions

- STEP 1

Boil the eggs for 6 mins, then quickly cool under cold running water and peel off the shells. Tip the lentils into a bowl with the onion, red pepper and balsamic vinegar. Mix well.

- STEP 2

Put the salad onto a serving dish, then pile the rocket on top. Drizzle with the oil, then halve the eggs and sit them on top of the salad.

Salmon meatballs in spicy lentil gravy

Ingredients

- 2 medium slices white bread

- 450g salmon fillet, cut into rough chucks

- 1 egg white

- 1 tbsp olive oil

For the spicy gravy

- 2 tbsp korma curry paste

- 1 small onion, finely chopped

- 2 red peppers, finely chopped

- 500g carton tomato passata

- 50g red lentils

Directions

• STEP 1

In a food processor, whizz the bread to fine crumbs. Set aside, then whizz the salmon. Add the crumbs and egg white, then pulse to combine. Season. Divide into 12 balls and chill for 30 mins. Can be frozen at this stage for up to 1 month.

• STEP 2

Heat oven to 200C/fan 180C/gas 6. Heat the oil in a non-stick frying pan. Add the fishballs and fry for 1-2 mins until lightly browned. Transfer to a baking tray, bake for 15 mins until golden.

• STEP 3

Wipe the pan, add korma paste and onion, and cook for 5 mins, stirring regularly. Add peppers and cook for 2 mins. Add passata and lentils, bring to the boil, then simmer for 20 mins. Coat fishballs in the gravy and serve.

Coriander roast chicken thighs with puy lentil salad

Ingredients

• 185g puy lentils

• 20g ginger, peeled

• 30g coriander, plus extra leaves to serve

• 1 tsp each garam masala and ground coriander

• ½ tsp ground cumin

• 2 large whole garlic cloves, plus 1 small clove, finely grated

• 2 tbsp lemon juice

- 150g pot plain bio yogurt

- 6 bone-in, skinless chicken thighs

- 1 tbsp fresh turmeric, finely grated

- 1 tbsp rapeseed or olive oil, plus 1 tsp

- 3 red onions (325g), thickly sliced

- 1 large red pepper and 1 large yellow pepper, deseeded and cut into chunks

- 400g cauliflower, cut into small florets

- 1 tsp cumin seeds

Directions

- STEP 1

Heat the oven to 220C/200C fan/ gas 7. Boil the lentils for 35-40 mins over a medium heat until tender.

• STEP 2

Meanwhile, put the ginger, fresh coriander, garam masala, the ground coriander, ground cumin and the 2 whole garlic cloves in a large bowl with half the lemon juice and 3 tbsp of the yogurt. Blitz using a hand blender until smooth. Use 4 tbsp of the mixture to coat the chicken thighs in a large bowl. Arrange the chicken on a baking tray in a single layer.

• STEP 3

Add the remaining yogurt to the remaining spice and herb mixture, along with the turmeric, 1 tsp oil, the grated garlic, 1 tbsp water and remaining lemon juice to taste. Set aside.

• STEP 4

Tip the onions, peppers and cauliflower into the bowl used for the chicken, and toss with 1 tbsp oil to coat in some of the spice mix. Spread the veg out on a baking tray, then put in the oven with the chicken for 30-35 mins until the chicken is cooked through.

• STEP 5

Remove the chicken and wrap in foil to keep it warm. Scatter the cumin seeds over the veg and return to the oven for 5 mins until golden.

• STEP 6

To serve, drain the lentils and put in a serving bowl with the roasted veg and the remaining turmeric yogurt. Gently toss together. Serve with the chicken (taking the meat off the bones), and scatter with the extra coriander

Fennel, cherry & goat's cheese salad with lentils

Ingredients

• 50g walnut halves or pieces

• 250g pack pre-cooked puy lentils

• 1 large fennel bulb, finely sliced, fronds reserved

• 140g cherries, halved and pitted (or small figs, halved)

• 1 tbsp red wine vinegar

• 2 tbsp extra virgin olive oil

• 1 tsp Dijon mustard

• ½ tsp clear honey

• ½ small pack tarragon, roughly chopped

• 100g pack soft goat's cheese (any kind will work, but ash-rolled looks a bit special), thickly sliced and halved

Directions

• STEP 1

Heat a dry frying pan over a low-medium heat. Add the walnuts and cook for 3 mins, stirring frequently, until they smell toasty and the skins are a deep golden brown. Set aside to cool.

• STEP 2

Heat the lentils following pack instructions, then tip into a large bowl and loosen with a fork. Tip the fennel and cherries on top.

• STEP 3

Whisk together the vinegar, oil, mustard, honey and tarragon, then season. Fold the dressing through the lentils, fennel and cherries, then scoop the salad onto a platter. Scatter with the cheese, walnuts and the reserved fennel fronds.

Prosciutto, kale & butter bean stew

Ingredients

• 80g pack prosciutto, torn into pieces

• 2 tbsp olive oil

• 1 fennel bulb, sliced

• 2 garlic clove, crushed

• 1 tsp chilli flakes

• 4 thyme sprigs

* 150ml white wine or chicken stock

* 2 x 400g cans butter beans

* 400g can cherry tomatoes

* 200g bag sliced kale

Directions

* STEP 1

Fry the prosciutto in a dry saucepan over a high heat until crisp, then remove half with a slotted spoon and set aside. Turn the heat down to low, pour in the oil and tip in the fennel with a pinch of salt. Cook for 5 mins until softened, then throw in the garlic, chilli flakes and thyme and cook for a further 2 mins, then pour in the wine or stock and bring to a simmer.

* STEP 2

Tip both cans of butter beans into the stew, along with their liquid, then add the tomatoes, season well and bring everything to a simmer. Cook, undisturbed, for 5 mins, then stir through the kale. Once wilted, ladle the stew into bowls, removing the thyme sprigs and topping each portion with the remaining prosciutto.

Feta & kale loaded sweet potato

Ingredients

• 2 sweet potatoes

• chickpeas, drained

• 1 red onion, thinly sliced

• 2tbsp red wine vinegar

• 30g feta, cut into small cubes

- 1 tsp caster sugar

- 1tbsp olive oil

- chilli flakes

- 100g kale

- 1tbsp pumpkin seeds, toasted

- rocket

Directions

- STEP 1

Heat oven to 200C/180C fan/gas 6. Prick the sweet potatoes all over with a fork, then put them in a roasting tin and roast for 40 mins. Add the chickpeas to the tray, then roast for 10 mins more, until the potatoes are completely tender and the chickpeas have crisped a little.

• STEP 2

Meanwhile, mix the onion with the vinegar and a pinch of sugar and salt, and set aside to quick pickle. In another bowl, marinate the feta with the oil and chilli flakes.

• STEP 3

When the potatoes are nearly cooked, cook the kale in a pan with 50ml water for 3 mins until wilted, then season to taste. Halve the potatoes, divide between two plates and top each with the kale, chickpeas, red onion (reserving the vinegar), marinated feta and pumpkin seeds. Toss the rocket with the reserved vinegar, then serve on the side.

Kale & quinoa patties

Ingredients

• 140g quinoa

• 500g hot vegetable stock

• 100g kale, stalks removed, leaves roughly chopped

• 3 tbsp olive oil

• 1 small onion, finely chopped

• 2 garlic cloves, crushed

• 75g fresh white breadcrumbs

• 2 medium eggs, beaten

• 50g sundried tomatoes, roughly chopped

• 100g goat's cheese, cut from a round log

• green salad, to serve (optional)

For the pesto

• ½ small pack basil, leaves only

• ½ small pack parsley, leaves only

• 2 garlic cloves, crushed

• 50g pine nuts, toasted

• 50g parmesan, grated

• 150g olive oil

• juice 1 lemon

Directions

• STEP 1

Put the quinoa in a saucepan and pour over the hot stock. Simmer for 18-20 mins over a gentle heat until the grains have fluffed up and the liquid has disappeared. Remove from the heat and allow to cool. Meanwhile, bring a large saucepan of water to the boil. Add the kale and simmer for 6-8 mins until cooked through. Drain, squeeze out any excess water and set aside.

• STEP 2

Put 1 tbsp olive oil in a small frying pan over a medium heat. Add the onion and cook for 2-3 mins until translucent. Add the garlic and cook for 1 min more. Tip the cooked quinoa into a bowl and add the kale, onion, garlic, breadcrumbs, egg and sundried tomatoes. Season well and mix to combine. Set aside.

• STEP 3

To make the pesto, put the basil, parsley, garlic, pine nuts and Parmesan in a small food processor. Pulse, slowly pouring in the oil, until you have a thick pesto. Squeeze in the lemon juice to loosen, then set aside.

• STEP 4

Gently heat 2 tbsp olive oil in a shallow frying pan. Using your hands, form the quinoa mixture into 8 round patties. Add to the frying pan and fry for 4-5 mins each side until crisp and golden.

• STEP 5

Heat the grill to high and put a slice of goat's cheese on top of each patty. Place under the grill to brown and melt the cheese slightly – this will take a matter of seconds, so keep an eye on them. Top each patty with a generous spoonful of pesto and serve with some fresh green leaves, if you like.

Kale & chorizo broth

Ingredients

• 3 tbsp olive oil

* 2 onions, finely chopped

* 4 garlic cloves, crushed

* 2-3 cooking chorizo sausages, sliced

* 4 large potatoes

* 1 ½l chicken stock

* 200g curly kale, finely shredded

Directions

* STEP 1

Heat 2 tbsp of the oil in a large saucepan. Add the onions, garlic and chorizo, then cook for 5 mins until soft. Throw in the potatoes and cook for a few mins more. Pour in the stock, season and bring to the boil. Cook everything for 10 mins until the potatoes are on the brink of collapse.

Use a masher to squash the potatoes into the soup, then bring back to the boil. Add the kale and cook for 5 mins until tender. Ladle the soup into bowls, then serve drizzled with the remaining olive oil.

Leek & butter bean soup with crispy kale & bacon

Ingredients

• 4 tsp olive oil

• 500g leeks, sliced

• 4 thyme sprigs, leaves picked

• 2 x 400g cans butter beans

• 500ml vegetable bouillon stock

- 2 tsp wholegrain mustard

- ½ small pack flat-leaf parsley

- 3 rashers streaky bacon

- 40g chopped kale, any tough stems removed

- 25g hazelnuts, roughly chopped

Directions

- STEP 1

Heat 1 tbsp oil in a large saucepan over a low heat. Add the leeks, thyme and seasoning. Cover and cook for 15 mins until softened, adding a splash of water if the leeks start to stick. Add the butter beans with the water from the cans, the stock and mustard. Bring to the boil and simmer for 3-4 mins until hot. Blend the soup in a food processor or with a stick blender, stir through the parsley and check the seasoning.

• STEP 2

Put the bacon in a large, non-stick frying pan over a medium heat. Cook for 3-4 mins until crispy, then set side to cool. Add the remaining 1 tsp oil to the pan, and tip in the kale and hazelnuts. Cook for 2 mins, stirring until the kale is wilted and crisping at the edges and the hazelnuts are toasted. Cut the bacon into small pieces, then stir into the kale mixture.

• STEP 3

Reheat the soup, adding a splash of water if it is too thick. Serve in bowls sprinkled with the bacon & kale mixture.

CHAPTER VII

NOURISHING DINNER RECIPES FOR SCLERODERMA

Homemade burgers with sweet potato wedges

Ingredients

For the burgers

• 1 tbsp olive oil, plus extra for drizzling

• 1 red onion, finely chopped

• 500g lean minced beef or turkey

• 1 egg

• 12 cream crackers, bashed to fine crumbs

• 2 tsp chilli paste

• 2 tsp garlic paste

• 1 tsp each, tomato ketchup and brown sauce

• 2 tbsp plain flour

• 6 hamburger rolls, toasted, to serve

• toppings of your choice (relish, chutney and salad
), to serve

For the wedges

• 4 sweet potatoes, cut into wedges

• 2 tbsp olive oil

• 1 tsp paprika

Directions

• STEP 1

Heat the oil in a frying pan and fry the onion for about 5 mins or until soft. Leave to cool slightly. When cool, put the onion in a large bowl with the mince, egg, bashed crackers, chilli, garlic, ketchup and brown sauce, and mix well to combine. Divide the mince into 6, roll into balls and flatten each into a nice fat burger.

• STEP 2

Put the flour on a plate, dab each burger to the flour on both sides, then transfer to a baking tray. Wrap with cling film and pop in the fridge for a couple of hours.

• STEP 3

Heat oven to 200C/180C fan/gas 6. To make the wedges, put the sweet potato on a baking tray and drizzle with olive oil. Sprinkle with paprika, season, then give them a good shake or shuffle around with your hands to make sure they're well coated. Roast for 30-40 mins depending on how crisp you like them. Make sure you give them a good shake a couple of times to ensure they cook evenly.

• STEP 4

When the wedges have been cooking for 10 mins, drizzle the burgers with a little olive oil and put them in the oven to cook with the wedges for the remaining 20-30 mins, flipping them halfway. 5 Serve the burgers in the rolls with your choice of toppings, and a good helping of wedges on the side.

Spicy turkey sweet potatoes

Ingredients

• 4 sweet potatoes

• 1 tbsp olive oil

• 1 onion, finely chopped

• 1 garlic clove, crushed

• 500g pack turkey thigh mince

• 500g carton passata

• 3 tbsp barbecue sauce

• ½ tsp cayenne pepper

• 4 tbsp soured cream

• ½ pack chives, finely snipped

Directions

• STEP 1

Heat oven to 200C/180C fan/gas 6. Prick the potatoes, place on a baking tray and bake for 45 mins or until really soft.

• STEP 2

Meanwhile, heat the oil in a frying pan, add the onion and cook gently for 8 mins until softened. Stir in the garlic, then tip in the mince and stir to break up. Cook over a high heat until any liquid has evaporated and the mince is browned, about 10 mins. Pour in the passata, then fill the carton a quarter full of water and tip that in too. Add the barbecue sauce and cayenne, then lower the heat and simmer gently for 15 mins, adding a little extra water if needed. Taste and season.

• STEP 3

When the potatoes are soft, split them down the centre and spoon the mince over the top. Add a dollop of soured cream and a sprinkling of chives

Roast squash with goat's cheese & puy lentils

Ingredients

• 800g delicata, acorn or butternut squash

• 4 tbsp rapeseed or olive oil

• 25g pumpkin seeds (or use the seeds from the pumpkin or squash you're using)

• 10 sage leaves

• 2 tbsp good-quality red wine vinegar

• 250g pouch cooked puy lentils

• 100g soft goat's cheese

• 4 amaretti biscuits

For the crispy kale

• 100g kale, rinsed, dried, thick stems removed and leaves torn into crisp-sized pieces

• ½ tbsp rapeseed or olive oil

• 1 tbsp white sesame seeds

• 1 tsp red chilli flakes

Procedure

• STEP 1

Heat oven to 160C/140C fan/gas 3. Toss the kale lightly in the oil, ½ tsp salt, sesame and chilli, massaging the leaves until coated with the oil and seasoning. Arrange the leaves in one layer in a roasting tin or baking tray – you might need to use more than one to keep them in an even layer. Roast for 15-20 mins until crisp and dry but not brown.

• STEP 2

Once dried, remove from the oven and turn the heat up to 200C/180C fan/gas 6. Halve the squash and scoop out the seeds. Wash the seeds to remove the sticky membrane, dry them with kitchen paper and set aside. Cut the squash into 1cm thick slices (don't worry about peeling them), and arrange on a baking sheet or in a roasting tin. Drizzle over 1 tbsp oil, season, then turn and drizzle with a little more oil. Season again and roast for 30-40 mins until tender and caramelising, turning halfway through. Remove from the oven.

• STEP 3

Heat the remaining oil in a non-stick frying pan over a medium to high heat until it's shimmering. Add the sage leaves and fry for 15-30 seconds, turning them once. Remove using tongs or a slotted spoon, place on kitchen paper and scatter with sea salt. Add the pumpkin seeds to the hot oil and fry for a few mins until puffed and crunchy. Drain the oil into a bowl and whisk with the red wine vinegar, a pinch of salt and freshly ground black pepper.

• STEP 4

Dress the lentils with half the dressing, then spoon onto the plates or serving platter. Arrange the crispy kale and squash on top, crumble over the goat's cheese, and drizzle over a bit more dressing. Finally, top with the fried seeds, and crumble over the amaretti biscuits and crispy sage leaves.

Chipolatas in apple gravy with parsnip colcannon

Ingredients

• 1 large potato, cut into chunks

• 4 parsnips, peeled and cut into chunks

• 8 chipolatas

• 50g butter

• 2 large red apples, cored and cut into slim wedges

• 8 spring onions, sliced, white and green parts separated

• 1 tbsp flour

• 1 beef or chicken stock cube

• 200g kale or Savoy cabbage, finely chopped

• 5ml milk

Procedure

• STEP 1

Put the potato and parsnips in a very large pan of water, bring to the boil and simmer for 10 mins or until the veg is tender. Meanwhile, cook the chipolatas in a large frying pan. When brown on all sides, transfer to a plate and add 25g butter to the pan. Add the apples and white part of the spring onions. Fry for 5-10 mins until softened and starting to caramelise.

• STEP 2

Add the kale to the boiling veg for the final few mins, before the potatoes and parsnips are completely soft. When the kale has wilted, drain the veg and leave to steam-dry in the colander. Heat the remaining butter in the same pan – don't worry about washing it out. Add the green parts of the spring onions and sizzle for a few mins to soften.

• STEP 3

Add the flour and stock cube to the apples and spring onions, stir for 1-2 mins, then add 400ml water, mixing to a smooth gravy. Return the sausages to the pan and bubble in the gravy for a few mins until heated through. Meanwhile, add the veg to the buttery spring onions, along with the milk and plenty of seasoning, and mash until the potato and parsnips are smooth. Serve the colcannon with the chipolatas and the gravy spooned over the top.

Salsa verde salmon with smashed chickpea salad

Ingredients

• 3 tsp olive oil

• 1 orange, zested and juiced

• 2 skin-on salmon fillets

• small bunch of parsley (including stalks), finely chopped

• ½ tbsp Dijon mustard

• 1 shallot or 1/2 small red onion, finely chopped

• ½ tbsp red wine vinegar

• 400g can chickpeas, drained and rinsed

• 2 roasted red peppers from a jar, drained and chopped

• 50g kale

Procedure

• STEP 1

Heat the grill to high. Whisk 1 tsp of the oil with the orange zest, a splash of the juice, lots of black pepper and a small pinch of salt. Put the salmon, skin-side down, on a non-stick baking tray and pour over the marinade. Leave to marinate at room temperature while you make the salsa.

• STEP 2

Put the parsley, mustard, half the shallot, the vinegar, 1 tsp oil, and the remaining orange juice in a small food processor and blitz to a thick sauce, adding a splash of water to loosen if needed.

• STEP 3

Heat the remaining oil in a frying pan and fry the remaining shallot for 5 mins. Stir in the chickpeas and some seasoning, turn up the heat and stir until the chickpeas are just starting to crisp. Mash roughly with a potato masher and stir in the roasted peppers and kale. Add a splash of water and cover with a lid until the kale is wilted. Keep warm over a low heat.

• STEP 4

Grill the salmon for 4-6 mins, or until cooked to your liking. Spoon half the chickpeas onto a plate, top with a salmon fillet (leaving the skin behind if you like), and spoon over some of the salsa verde. Leave the remaining salmon fillet to cool to use in the lunchbox, see tip below.

RECIPE TIPS

FOR THE LEFTOVER LUNCHBOX

Put the leftover chickpea salad into a lunchbox with some halved cherry tomatoes. Flake over the leftover salmon, and top with the remaining salsa verde. Chill overnight, or until ready to eat.

Veggie tahini lentils

Ingredients

• 50g tahini

• zest and juice 1 lemon

- 2 tbsp olive oil

- 1 red onion, thinly sliced

- 1 garlic clove, crushed

- 1 yellow pepper, thinly sliced

- 200g green beans, trimmed and halved

- 1 courgette, sliced into half moons

- 100g shredded kale

- 250g pack pre-cooked puy lentils

Procedure

- STEP 1

In a jug, mix the tahini with the zest and juice of the lemon and 50ml of cold water to make a runny dressing. Season to taste, then set aside.

• STEP 2

Heat the oil in a wok or large frying pan over a medium-high heat. Add the red onion, along with a pinch of salt, and fry for 2 mins until starting to soften and colour. Add the garlic, pepper, green beans and courgette and fry for 5 min, stirring frequently.

• STEP 3

Tip in the kale, lentils and the tahini dressing. Keep the pan on the heat for a couple of mins, stirring everything together until the kale is wilted and it's all coated in the creamy dressing.

Kale & apple soup with walnuts

Ingredients

• 8 walnut halves, broken into pieces

* 1 onion, finely chopped

* 2 carrots, coarsely grated

* 2 red apples, unpeeled and finely chopped

* 1 tbsp cider vinegar

* 500ml reduced-salt vegetable stock

* 200g kale, roughly chopped

* 20g pack of dried apple crisps (optional)

Procedure

* STEP 1

In a dry, non-stick frying pan, cook the walnut pieces for 2-3 mins until toasted, turning frequently so they don't burn. Take off the heat and allow to cool.

* STEP 2

Put the onion, carrots, apples, vinegar and stock in a large saucepan and bring to the boil. Reduce the heat and simmer for 10 mins, stirring occasionally.

• STEP 3

Once the onion is translucent and the apples start to soften, add the kale and simmer for an additional 2 mins. Carefully transfer to a blender or liquidiser and blend until very smooth. Pour into bowls and serve topped with the toasted walnuts, and a sprinkling of apple crisps, if you like.

Mushroom risotto

Ingredients

• 50g dried porcini mushrooms

• 1 vegetable stock cube

* 2 tbsp olive oil

* 1 onion, finely chopped

* 2 garlic cloves, finely chopped

* 250g pack chestnut mushrooms, chopped

* 300g risotto rice, such as arborio

* 1 x 175ml glass white wine

* 25g butter

* handful parsley leaves, chopped

* 50g parmesan or Grana Padano, freshly grated

Directions

* STEP 1

Put 50g dried porcini mushrooms into a large bowl
and pour over 1 litre boiling water. Soak for 20 mins,

then drain into a bowl, discarding the last few tbsp of liquid left in the bowl.

• STEP 2

Crumble 1 vegetable stock cube into the mushroom liquid, then squeeze the mushrooms gently to remove any liquid.

• STEP 3

Heat 2 tbsp olive oil in a shallow saucepan or deep frying pan over a medium flame. Add 1 finely chopped onion and 2 finely chopped garlic cloves, then fry for about 5 mins until soft.

• STEP 4

Stir in 250g chopped chestnut mushrooms and the dried mushrooms, season with salt and pepper and continue to cook for 8 mins until the fresh mushrooms have softened.

• STEP 5

Tip 300g risotto rice into the pan and cook for 1 min. Pour over a 175ml glass of white wine and let it bubble to nothing so the alcohol evaporates.

• STEP 6

Keep the pan over a medium heat and pour in a quarter of the mushroom stock. Simmer the rice, stirring often, until the rice has absorbed all the liquid.

• STEP 7

Add about the same amount of stock again and continue to simmer and stir - it should start to become creamy, plump and tender. By the time the final quarter of stock is added, the rice should be almost cooked.

• STEP 8

Continue stirring until the rice is cooked. If the rice is still undercooked, add a splash of water. Take the pan off the heat, add 25g butter and scatter over 25g grated parmesan or Grana Padano cheese and half a handful of chopped parsley leaves.

• STEP 9

Cover and leave for a few mins so that the rice can take up any excess liquid as it cools a bit. Give the risotto a final stir, spoon into bowls and scatter with the remaining 25g grated cheese and the remaining chopped parsley leaves.

Chinese chicken curry

Ingredients

- 4 skinless chicken breasts, cut into chunks (or use thighs or drumsticks)

- 2 tsp cornflour

- 1 onion, diced

- 2 tbsp rapeseed oil

- 1 garlic clove, crushed

- 2 tsp curry powder

- 1 tsp turmeric

- ½ tsp ground ginger

- pinch sugar

- 400ml chicken stock

- 1 tsp soy sauce

- handful frozen peas

- rice to serve

Directions

- STEP 1

Toss the chicken pieces in the cornflour and season well. Set them aside.

- STEP 2

Fry the onion in half of the oil in a wok on a low to medium heat, until it softens – about 5-6 minutes – then add the garlic and cook for a minute. Stir in the spices and sugar and cook for another minute, then add the stock and soy sauce, bring to a simmer and cook for 20 minutes. Tip everything into a blender and blitz until smooth.

- STEP 3

Wipe out the pan and fry the chicken in the remaining oil until it is browned all over. Tip the sauce back into the pan and bring everything to a simmer, stir in the peas and cook for 5 minutes. Add a little water if you need to thin the sauce. Serve with rice.

Moroccan-style chickpea soup

Ingredients

• 1 tbsp olive oil

• 1 onion, chopped

• 2 celery sticks, chopped

• 2 tsp ground cumin

• 600ml hot vegetable stock

• 400g can chopped plum tomatoes with garlic

* 400g can chickpeas, rinsed and drained

* 100g frozen broad beans

* zest and juice ½ lemon

* large handful coriander or parsley and flatbread, to serve

Directions

* STEP 1

Heat the oil in a large saucepan, then fry the onion and celery gently for 10 mins until softened, stirring frequently. Tip in the cumin and fry for another min.

* STEP 2

Turn up the heat, then add the stock, tomatoes and chickpeas, plus a good grind of black pepper. Simmer for 8 mins. Throw in broad beans and lemon juice, cook for a further 2 mins. Season to taste, then top with a sprinkling of lemon zest and chopped herbs. Serve with flatbread.

Honey chicken

Ingredients

• 4 chicken breasts (about 600g), trimmed and cut into 2-3cm cubes

• 2 tbsp plain flour

• 40g piece of ginger, peeled and finely grated

• 4 garlic cloves, finely chopped

• 6 tbsp soy sauce

• 5 tbsp honey

• ½-1 lemon, juiced

• 1 tbsp sunflower, vegetable, rice bran or rapeseed oil

• cooked rice and steamed broccoli, to serve (optional)

Directions

• STEP 1

Tip the chicken into a bowl, sprinkle over the flour and some seasoning and toss until the chicken is evenly coated.

• STEP 2

Combine the ginger, garlic, soy, honey and half the lemon juice in a bowl. Heat the oil in a large frying pan or wok over a high heat and fry the chicken for 3-4 mins until lightly golden. Tip in the honey sauce and stir-fry for 10 mins, or until the chicken is cooked through and the sauce has reduced enough to coat the back of a spoon. Taste for seasoning and squeeze over the remaining lemon juice, if needed, then serve with rice and steamed broccoli, if you like.

Fajita chicken rice bowl with burnt lime

Ingredients

• 2 large chicken breasts

• 2 peppers, sliced

• 2 red onions, sliced

• 200g baby corn

• 3 tsp chipotle chilli paste

• 1 lime, zested, then halved

• 2 tsp vegetable oil

* 400g can black beans, drained

* 15g coriander, roughly chopped

* 400g cooked brown rice

* 4 tbsp salsa, to serve

Directions

* STEP 1

Heat the oven to 220C/200C fan/gas 7 and line a large baking tray with baking parchment. Arrange the chicken, peppers, red onions and baby corn on the tray, and spoon over the chipotle paste. Season, then toss to combine. Put the lime halves on the tray, cut-side down, then drizzle the oil over the chicken and veg. Roast for 20 mins, or until everything is cooked through.

* STEP 2

Meanwhile, warm the beans in a small pan over a low heat, and season. Mix the beans with half the coriander and the lime zest, then squeeze over the juice of the roasted lime. Slice the chicken thinly on the diagonal and divide between four bowls along with the veg and brown rice. Sprinkle over the remaining coriander and serve with the salsa.

Ginger chicken udon noodles

Ingredients

• 1 tsp sunflower oil

• 3 boneless, skinless chicken thighs, diced

• ¼ white cabbage, finely sliced

• 25g ginger, peeled and finely grated

• 1 red chilli (deseeded if you like), finely chopped

• 1 tbsp low-salt soy sauce

• 2 tsp rice vinegar

• 2 tsp mirin

• 100g ready-to-eat beansprouts

• 3 spring onions, finely sliced

• 300g straight-to-wok udon noodles

• small handful of coriander, finely chopped

• 1 tbsp pickled ginger (optional)

Directions

• STEP 1

Heat the oil in a large, deep frying pan over a medium-high heat and, once hot, stir-fry the chicken and cabbage for 5-7 mins until browned and almost cooked through. Add the ginger and chilli, and cook for a few minutes more until fragrant.

• STEP 2

Add the remaining Ingredients, except the coriander and pickled ginger, and fry until the chicken is cooked and the noodles are tender, about 1-2 mins more. Season, adding more soy, vinegar or mirin, if you like. Top with the coriander and pickled ginger, if using.

Tuna, asparagus & white bean salad

Ingredients

• 1 large bunch asparagus

• 2 x cans tuna steaks in water, drained

• 2 x cans cannellini beans in water, drained

- 1 red onion, very finely chopped

- 2 tbsp capers

- 1 tbsp olive oil

- 1 tbsp red wine vinegar

- 2 tbsp tarragon, finely chopped

Directions

- STEP 1

Cook the asparagus in a large pan of boiling water for 4-5 mins until tender. Drain well, cool under running water, then cut into finger-length pieces. Toss together the tuna, beans, onion, capers and asparagus in a large serving bowl.

- STEP 2

Mix the oil, vinegar and tarragon together, then pour over the salad. Chill until ready to serve.

Spanish rice & prawn one-pot

Ingredients

• 1 onion, sliced

• 1 red and 1 green pepper, deseeded and sliced

• 50g chorizo, sliced

• 2 garlic cloves, crushed

• 1 tbsp olive oil

• 250g easy cook basmati rice (we used Tilda)

• 400g can chopped tomato

• 200g raw, peeled prawns, defrosted if frozen

Directions

• STEP 1

Boil the kettle. In a non-stick frying or shallow pan with a lid, fry the onion, peppers, chorizo and garlic in the oil over a high heat for 3 mins. Stir in the rice and chopped tomatoes with 500ml boiling water, cover, then cook over a high heat for 12 mins.

• STEP 2

Uncover, then stir – the rice should be almost tender. Stir in the prawns, with a splash more water if the rice is looking dry, then cook for another min until the prawns are just pink and rice tender.

CHAPTER VIII

NOURISHING SOUP RECIPES FOR SCLERODERMA

Corn & split pea chowder

Ingredients

• 200g dried yellow split peas

• 3 celery sticks (about 160g), sliced

• 1 thyme sprig, plus 1 tbsp thyme leaves

• 2 onions (350g), halved and sliced

• 1 tbsp rapeseed oil

• 50g ginger, finely grated

• 2 red chillies, deseeded and sliced

• 3 garlic cloves, chopped

• 1 large green pepper, chopped into small pieces

• 1 potato (about 215g), unpeeled, cut into 1-2cm pieces

• 2 tbsp vegetable bouillon powder

• 320g frozen sweetcorn

• 150g coconut yogurt

Instructions

• STEP 1

Tip the split peas, celery and thyme sprig into a medium pan with 1 litre of boiling water, bring back to the boil and simmer, covered, for 25 mins.

• STEP 2

Meanwhile, fry the onion in the oil in a large pan for 10 mins. Stir in the ginger, chilli and garlic. Tip in the pepper and potato, and pour in ½ litre boiling water with the bouillon and remaining thyme. Tip in the split pea mixture and corn, bring to the boil, then cover and simmer for 30-35 mins until the veg is tender.

• STEP 3

Remove the thyme sprig. Take out a third of the veg, then purée the rest in the pan with a hand blender (or use a potato masher). Return the veg to the pan with the yogurt, and stir well. Serve when done.

Broccoli and kale green soup

Ingredients

• 500ml stock, made by mixing 1 tbsp bouillon powder and boiling water in a jug

• 1 tbsp sunflower oil

• 2 garlic cloves, sliced

• thumb-sized piece ginger, sliced

• ½ tsp ground coriander

• 3cm/1in piece fresh turmeric root, peeled and grated, or 1/2 tsp ground turmeric

• pinch of pink Himalayan salt

• 200g courgettes, roughly sliced

• 85g broccoli

• 100g kale, chopped

• 1 lime, zested and juiced

• small pack parsley, roughly chopped, reserving a few whole leaves to serve

Instructions

• STEP 1

Put the oil in a deep pan, add the garlic, ginger, coriander, turmeric and salt, fry on a medium heat for 2 mins, then add 3 tbsp water to give a bit more moisture to the spices.

• STEP 2

Add the courgettes, making sure you mix well to coat the slices in all the spices, and continue cooking for 3 mins. Add 400ml stock and leave to simmer for 3 mins.

• STEP 3

Add the broccoli, kale and lime juice with the rest of the stock. Leave to cook again for another 3-4 mins until all the vegetables are soft.

• STEP 4

Take off the heat and add the chopped parsley. Pour everything into a blender and blend on high speed until smooth. It will be a beautiful green with bits of dark speckled through (which is the kale). Garnish with lime zest and parsley.

Fresh tomato soup with cheesy cornbread

Ingredients

For the bread

• 40g wholemeal self-raising flour

- 85g ground polenta

- 1 tsp baking powder

- 40g mature cheddar, finely grated

- 1 tsp smoked paprika

- 3 spring onions (35g), finely sliced

- 1 green chilli, deseeded, finely sliced

- 1 large egg

- 125ml milk

For the soup

- 2 tsp rapeseed oil

- 3-5 sticks celery (165g), finely chopped

- 2 onions, chopped

• 4 carrots (320g), diced

• 325g floury potatoes, grated

• 500g tomatoes, chopped

• 4 tsp vegetable bouillon powder made up to 1 1/2 litre with boiling water

• 3 tbsp tomato purée

• 2 large garlic cloves, finely grated

• flat-leaf parsley, chopped, to serve

Instructions

• STEP 1

First, make the bread. Heat oven to 200C/180C fan/gas 6 and line the base of a non-stick 500g loaf tin with baking parchment. Tip the flour, polenta and baking powder into a bowl with half the cheese, the paprika, onions and chilli, then toss together. Add the egg and milk and mix well. Turn out into the tin and top with the remaining cheese. Bake for 20-25 mins until golden and a skewer inserted into the centre comes out clean.

• STEP 2

To make the soup, heat the oil in a large pan and fry the celery, onion and carrots for 10 mins until softened. Add the potatoes, tomatoes, bouillon, tomato purée and garlic, then stir well. Cover with a lid and cook for 20 mins.

• STEP 3

Remove from the heat and blitz until smooth with a hand blender. Spoon the soup into two bowls and scatter with parsley.

Summer pistou

Ingredients

- 1 tbsp rapeseed oil

- 2 leeks, finely sliced

- 1 large courgette, finely diced

- 1l boiling vegetable stock (made from scratch or with reduced-salt bouillon)

- 400g can cannellini or haricot beans, drained

- 200g green beans, chopped

- 3 tomatoes, chopped

- 3 garlic cloves, finely chopped

- small pack basil

• 40g freshly grated parmesan

Instructions

• STEP 1

Heat the oil in a large pan and fry the leeks and courgette for 5 mins to soften. Pour in the stock, add three-quarters of the haricot beans with the green beans, half the tomatoes, and simmer for 5-8 mins until the vegetables are tender.

• STEP 2

Meanwhile, blitz the remaining beans and tomatoes, the garlic and basil in a food processor (or in a bowl with a stick blender) until smooth, then stir in the Parmesan. Stir the sauce into the soup, cook for 1 min, then ladle half into bowls or pour into a flask for a packed lunch. Chill the remainder. Will keep for a couple of days.

Spinach soup

Ingredients

• 25g butter

• 1 bunch spring onions, chopped

• 1 leek (about 120g), sliced

• 2 small sticks celery (about 85g), sliced

• 1 small potato (about 200g), peeled and diced

• ½ tsp ground black pepper

• 1l stock (made with two chicken or vegetable stock cubes)

• 2 x 200-235g bags spinach

• 150g half-fat crème fraîche

Instructions

• STEP 1

Heat the butter in a large saucepan. Add the spring onions, leek, celery and potato. Stir and put on the lid. Sweat for 10 minutes, stirring a couple of times.

• STEP 2

Pour in the stock and cook for 10 – 15 minutes until the potato is soft.

• STEP 3

Add the spinach and cook for a couple of minutes until wilted. Use a hand blender to blitz to a smooth soup.

• STEP 4

Stir in the crème fraîche. Reheat and serve.

Red lentil soup

Ingredients

• 1 white onion, finely sliced

• 2 tsp olive oil

• 3 garlic cloves, sliced

• 2 carrots, scrubbed and diced

• 85g red lentils

• 1 vegetable stock cube, crumbled

• generous sprigs parsley, chopped (about 2 tbsp) plus a few extra leaves

Instructions

• STEP 1

Put the kettle on to boil while you finely slice the onion. Heat the oil in a medium pan, add the onion and fry for 2 mins while you slice the garlic and dice the carrots. Add them to the pan, and cook briefly over the heat.

• STEP 2

Pour in 1 litre of the boiling water from the kettle, stir in the lentils and stock cube, then cover the pan and cook over a medium heat for 15 mins until the lentils are tender. Take off the heat and stir in the parsley. Ladle into bowls, and scatter with extra parsley leaves, if you like.

Courgette, pea & pesto soup

Ingredients

• 1 tbsp olive oil

• 1 garlic clove, sliced

• 500g courgettes, quartered lengthways and chopped

• 200g frozen peas

• 400g can cannellini beans, drained and rinsed

• 1l hot vegetable stock

• 2 tbsp basil pesto, or vegetarian alternative

Instructions

• STEP 1

Heat the oil in a large saucepan. Cook the garlic for a few seconds, then add the courgettes and cook for 3 mins until they start to soften. Stir in the peas and cannellini beans, pour on the hot stock and cook for a further 3 mins.

• STEP 2

Stir the pesto through the soup with some seasoning, then ladle into bowls and serve with crusty brown bread, if you like. Or pop in a flask to take to work.

Cucumber, pea & lettuce soup

Ingredients

• 1 tsp rapeseed oil

• small bunch spring onions, roughly chopped

• 1 cucumber, roughly chopped

• 1 large round lettuce, roughly chopped

• 225g frozen peas

• 4 tsp vegetable bouillon

• 4 tbsp bio yogurt (optional)

• 4 slices rye bread

Instructions

• STEP 1

Boil 1.4 litres water in a kettle. Heat the oil in a large non-stick frying pan and cook the spring onions for 5 mins, stirring frequently, or until softened. Add the cucumber, lettuce and peas, then pour in the boiled water. Stir in the bouillon, cover and simmer for 10 mins or until the vegetables are soft but still bright green.

• STEP 2

Blitz the mixture with a hand blender until smooth. Serve hot or cold, topped with yogurt (if you like), with rye bread alongside.

Chicken & sweetcorn soup

Ingredients

- 1 chicken carcass

- 4 thin slices fresh ginger, plus 1 tbsp finely grated

- 2 onions, quartered

- 3 garlic cloves, finely grated

- 2 tsp apple cider vinegar

- 325g can sweetcorn

- 3 spring onions, whites thinly sliced, greens sliced at an angle

- 100g cooked chicken, shredded

- 2 tsp tamari

• 2 eggs, beaten

• few drops sesame oil, to serve (optional)

Instructions

• STEP 1

Boil a large kettle of water. Break the carcass into a big non-stick pan and add the ginger slices, onion and two-thirds of the garlic. Cook, stirring, for about 2 mins – the meat will stick to the base of the pan, but this will add to the flavour. Pour in 1.5 litres of boiling water, stir in the vinegar, then cover and simmer for 2 hrs.

• STEP 2

Put a large sieve over a bowl and pour through the contents of the pan. Measure the liquid in the bowl – you want around 450ml. If you have too much, return to the pan and boil with the lid off to reduce it. Transfer the onion from the sieve to a bowl with three-quarters of the sweetcorn. Blitz until smooth with a hand blender.

• STEP 3

Return the broth to the pan, and tip in the puréed corn, remaining sweetcorn and garlic, the grated ginger, the whites of the spring onions and the chicken. Simmer for 5 mins, then stir in the tamari. Turn off the heat, and quickly drizzle in the egg, stirring a little to create egg threads. Season with pepper, then ladle into the bowls. Top with the spring onion greens and a few drops of sesame oil, if using.

Moroccan spiced cauliflower & almond soup

Ingredients

* 1 large cauliflower

* 2 tbsp olive oil

* ½ tsp each ground cinnamon, cumin and coriander

* 2 tbsp harissa paste, plus extra drizzle

* 1l hot vegetable or chicken stock

* 50g toasted flaked almond, plus extra to serve

Instructions

* STEP 1

Cut the cauliflower into small florets. Fry olive oil, ground cinnamon, cumin and coriander and harissa paste for 2 mins in a large pan. Add the cauliflower, stock and almonds. Cover and cook for 20 mins until the cauliflower is tender. Blend soup until smooth, then serve with an extra drizzle of harissa and a sprinkle of toasted almonds.

Broccoli & stilton soup

Ingredients

• 2 tbsp rapeseed oil

• 1 onion, finely chopped

• 1 stick celery, sliced

• 1 leek, sliced

• 1 medium potato, diced

• 1 knob butter

• 1l low salt or homemade chicken or vegetable stock

• 1 head broccoli, roughly chopped

• 140g stilton, or other blue cheese, crumbled

Instructions

• STEP 1

Heat 2 tbsp rapeseed oil in a large saucepan and then add 1 finely chopped onion. Cook on a medium heat until soft. Add a splash of water if the onion starts to catch.

• STEP 2

Add 1 sliced celery stick, 1 sliced leek, 1 diced medium potato and a knob of butter. Stir until melted, then cover with a lid. Allow to sweat for 5 minutes then remove the lid.

• STEP 3

Pour in 1l of chicken or vegetable stock and add any chunky bits of stalk from 1 head of broccoli. Cook for 10-15 minutes until all the vegetables are soft.

• STEP 4

Add the rest of the roughly chopped broccoli and cook for a further 5 minutes.

• STEP 5

Carefully transfer to a blender and blitz until smooth.

• STEP 6

Stir in 140g crumbled stilton, allowing a few lumps to remain. Season with black pepper and serve.

Mushroom & potato soup

Ingredients

- 1 tbsp rapeseed oil

- 2 large onions, halved and thinly sliced

- 20g dried porcini mushrooms

- 3 tsp vegetable bouillon powder

- 300g chestnut mushrooms, chopped

- 3 garlic cloves, finely grated

- 300g potato, finely diced

- 2 tsp fresh thyme

- 4 carrots, finely diced

- 2 tbsp chopped parsley

- 8 tbsp bio yogurt

- 55g walnut pieces

Instructions

• STEP 1

Heat the oil in a large pan. Tip in the onions and fry for 10 mins until golden. Meanwhile, pour 1.2 litres boiling water over the dried mushrooms and stir in the bouillon.

• STEP 2

Add the fresh mushrooms and garlic to the pan with the potatoes, thyme and carrots, and continue to fry until the mushrooms soften and start to brown.

• STEP 3

Pour in the dried mushrooms and stock, cover the pan and leave to simmer for 20 mins. Stir in the parsley and plenty of pepper. Ladle into bowls and serve each portion topped with 2 tbsp yogurt and a quarter of the walnuts. The rest can be chilled and reheated the next day.

Summer carrot, tarragon & white bean soup

Ingredients

• 1 tbsp rapeseed oil

• 2 large leeks, well washed, halved lengthways and finely sliced

• 700g carrots, chopped

• 1.4l hot reduced-salt vegetable bouillon (we used Marigold)

• 4 garlic cloves, finely grated

• 2 x 400g cans cannellini beans in water

• ⅔ small pack tarragon, leaves roughly chopped

Instructions

• STEP 1

Heat the oil over a medium heat in a large pan and fry the leeks and carrots for 5 mins to soften.

• STEP 2

Pour over the stock, stir in the garlic, the beans with their liquid, and three-quarters of the tarragon, then cover and simmer for 15 mins or until the veg is just tender. Stir in the remaining tarragon before serving.

Tomato soup

Ingredients

• 1-1.25kg/2lb 4oz-2lb 12oz ripe tomatoes

• 1 medium onion

• 1 small carrot

• 1 celery stick

• 2 tbsp olive oil

• 2 squirts of tomato purée (about 2 tsp)

• a good pinch of sugar

• 2 bay leaves

• 1.2 litres/2 pints hot vegetable stock (made with boiling water and 4 rounded tsp bouillon powder or 2 stock cubes)

Instructions

• STEP 1

First, prepare your vegetables. You need 1-1.25kg/2lb 4oz-2lb 12oz ripe tomatoes. If the tomatoes are on their vines, pull them off. The green stalky bits should come off at the same time, but if they don't, just pull or twist them off afterwards. Throw the vines and green bits away and wash the tomatoes. Now cut each tomato into quarters and slice off any hard cores (they don't soften during cooking and you'd get hard bits in the soup at the end). Peel 1 medium onion and 1 small carrot and chop them into small pieces. Chop 1 celery stick roughly the same size.

• STEP 2

Spoon 2 tbsp olive oil into a large heavy-based pan and heat it over a low heat. Hold your hand over the pan until you can feel the heat rising from the oil, then tip in the onion, carrot and celery and mix them together with a wooden spoon. Still with the heat low, cook the vegetables until they're soft and faintly coloured. This should take about 10 minutes and you should stir them two or three times so they cook evenly and don't stick to the bottom of the pan.

• STEP 3

Holding the tube over the pan, squirt in about 2 tsp of tomato purée, then stir it around so it turns the vegetables red. Shoot the tomatoes in off the chopping board, sprinkle in a good pinch of sugar and grind in a little black pepper. Tear 2 bay leaves into a few pieces and throw them into the pan. Stir to mix everything together, put the lid on the pan and let the tomatoes stew over a low heat for 10 minutes until they shrink down in the pan and their juices flow nicely. From time to time, give the pan a good shake – this will keep everything well mixed.

• STEP 4

Slowly pour in the 1.2 litres/2 pints of hot stock (made with boiling water and 4 rounded tsp bouillon powder or 2 stock cubes), stirring at the same time to mix it with the vegetables. Turn up the heat as high as it will go and wait until everything is bubbling, then turn the heat down to low again and put the lid back on the pan. Cook gently for 25 minutes, stirring a couple of times. At the end of cooking the tomatoes will have broken down and be very slushy-looking.

• STEP 5

Remove the pan from the heat, take the lid off and stand back for a few seconds or so while the steam escapes, then fish out the pieces of bay leaf and throw them away. Ladle the soup into your blender until it's about three-quarters full, fit the lid on tightly and turn the machine on full. Blitz until the soup's smooth (stop the machine and lift the lid to check after about 30 seconds), then pour the puréed soup into a large bowl. Repeat with the soup that's left in the pan. (The soup may now be frozen for up to three months. Defrost before reheating.)

• STEP 6

Pour the puréed soup back into the pan and reheat it over a medium heat for a few minutes, stirring occasionally until you can see bubbles breaking gently on the surface. Taste a spoonful and add a pinch or two of salt if you think the soup needs it, plus more pepper and sugar if you like. If the colour's not a deep enough red for you, plop in another teaspoon of tomato purée and stir until it dissolves. Ladle into bowls and serve. Or sieve and serve chilled with some cream swirled in.

CHAPTER IX

BEFORE YOU LEAVE, A FINAL WORD!

Lifestyle and home remedies

You can take a number of steps to help manage your symptoms of scleroderma:

• **Stay active**. Exercise keeps your body flexible, improves circulation and eases stiffness. Range-of-motion exercises can help keep your skin and joints flexible. This is always very important, especially early in the disease course.

• **Protect your skin**. Take good care of dry or stiff skin by using lotion and sunscreen regularly. Avoid hot baths and showers and exposure to strong soaps and household chemicals, which can irritate and further dry out your skin.

• **Don't smoke**. Nicotine causes blood vessels to contract, making Raynaud's phenomenon worse. Smoking also can cause permanent narrowing of the blood vessels and cause or worsen lung problems. Quitting smoking can be difficult. Ask your healthcare professional for help.

• **Manage heartburn**. Avoid foods that give you heartburn or gas. Also avoid late-night meals. Elevate the head of your bed to keep stomach acid from backing up into your esophagus as you sleep. Antacids may help relieve symptoms.

• **Protect yourself from the cold.** Wear warm mittens for protection anytime your hands are exposed to cold — even when you reach into a freezer. It also is important to keep your core body temperature warm to help prevent Raynaud's phenomenon. When you're outside in the cold, wear warm boots, cover your face and head, and wear layers of warm clothing.

Coping and support

As is true with other chronic diseases, living with scleroderma can cause you to feel anxious or worried. Here are some ideas to help you even out your feelings:

• Maintain your typical daily activities as best you can.

• Pace yourself and be sure to get the rest that you need.

• Stay connected with friends and family.

• Continue to pursue hobbies that you enjoy and are able to do.

Keep in mind that your physical health can have a direct impact on your mental health. People with chronic illnesses can feel denial, anger and frustration.

At times, you may need additional tools to deal with your emotions. Mental health professionals, such as therapists or behavior psychologists, may be able to help you put things in perspective. They also can help you develop coping skills, including relaxation techniques.

Joining a support group, where you can share experiences and feelings with other people, is often a good approach. Ask your healthcare team what support groups are available in your community.

Living with Scleroderma

Scleroderma can impact your life in many ways. In addition to following your doctor's treatment plan, here are a few things you can do to manage your symptoms, for instance:

• Follow a diet and exercise plan that's healthy for you.

• Eat small, frequent meals. After you eat, stay upright for 3 hours and try to avoid slouching.

• Eat moist, soft foods, and chew them well. If your doctor recommends a specific diet, follow that.

• Avoid caffeine, alcohol, and tobacco.

• Drink plenty of water and stay hydrated.

• Rest and avoid intense physical activity when you don't feel well.

• Avoid cold or wet environments, if you can, to help control Raynaud's symptoms.

• Protect your skin by wearing the right clothes for your environment and sunscreen when you're outside. Treat dry, itchy skin with lotions and moisturizers.

• Visit your dentist regularly for cleaning and checkups.

• Create a support network of friends and family.

• Improve your stress and mental health through counseling or group therapy.